PREGNANCY WEIGHT MANAGEMENT

Before, During, After

THERESA FRANCIS-CHEUNG

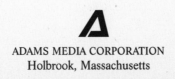
ADAMS MEDIA CORPORATION
Holbrook, Massachusetts

Published by
Adams Media Corporation
260 Center Street, Holbrook, MA 02343. U.S.A.
www.adamsmedia.com

ISBN: 1-58062-333-6

Printed in Canada

J I H G F E D C B

Library of Congress Cataloging-in-Publication Data
Francis-Cheung, Theresa
Pregnancy Weight Management: before, during, after / Theresa Francis-Cheung.
p.   cm.
Includes index.
ISBN 1-58062-333-6
1. Pregnancy—Nutritional aspects—Popular works.
2. Pregnant women—Weight gain—Popular works. 3. Physical fitness for women—
Popular works. 4. Weight loss—Popular works. I. Title
RG559 .F73   2000
618.2'4   00-038570

Pregnancy Weight Management does not purport to render medical
advice. Every pregnant woman should consult her professional health
care provider for such advice.

Interior illustrations by Roberta Collier-Morales
Cover photo by Norbert Schäfer/The Stock Market

This book is available at quantity discounts for bulk purchases.
For information, call 1-800-872-5627.

Contents

Part One
Looking Pregnant, Feeling Fat

Part Two
Weight Management During Pregnancy

List of Illustrations

Foreword

by Dr. Arlene Jacobs, Obstetrician,
Gynecologist, and Infertility Specialist at
the Plano Medical Center in Plano, Texas

AS A DOCTOR I SEE PREGNANT WOMEN MONTHLY AND THEN WEEKLY. WITH our culture's obsession with thinness I know that a tremendous source of anxiety for pregnant women is their expanding waistline, a changing body image, and never getting back to their prepregnancy weight. I also know how discouraging it can be for women who still have a lot of weight to lose at their six-week postpartum check up.

There is a need for more information and advice about weight management during pregnancy and postpartum. Far too many women don't really understand what a healthy weight gain during pregnancy is, what "eating for two" means, and what to realistically expect in terms of weight loss in the postpartum period.

Diet, exercise, and weight management are always important. They become even more important when a woman has a baby. *Pregnancy Weight Management* is a reference guide for new moms. It discusses weight management before conception, during pregnancy, and in the first weeks, months, and years of motherhood. Common-sense advice based on personal experience and medical research is offered. The book is designed to help women through the challenging and exciting transition that is motherhood—when not just your body, but your whole life changes.

Acknowledgments

MY THANKS TO ALL THE MANY PEOPLE WHO HELPED PROVIDE INFORMATION about pregnancy and postpartum weight management for this book. In particular I thank Dr. Arlene Jacobs, obstetrician, gynecologist, and infertility specialist at the Plano Medical Center in Texas, for permission to quote her and for her invaluable advice, comments, and help with research while I was writing the book. Thanks also to Dr. James Douglas, reproductive endocrinologist and infertility specialist at the medical center in Plano, Texas, and to Dr. Priscilla Stuckey for her invaluable help with the manuscript in the formative and developmental editing stage. I would also like to express my gratitude to all the moms who talked to me about their bodies and for the insight they gave me. Their stories are in this book, with names and places changed to preserve identity. They provided much of the incentive to write this book. I am also indebted to the staff at Adams Media, in particular Cheryl Kimball for her help, advice, encouragement, and insight throughout.

Thanks also to my brother, Terry, and for the support of friends and family. Special gratitude to my husband, Ray, not only for his contributory chapter but for his patience, support, enthusiasm, and love while I completed this project. And finally, thanks to my son, Robert, for the joy he brings into my life.

Introduction

I CAN'T REMEMBER A TIME WHEN I DIDN'T WORRY ABOUT HOW MUCH I weighed. When I got pregnant, I knew that weight gain was inevitable. I was a little frightened. I had no idea how I was going to cope.

In the first trimester I anxiously watched the scale. If I gained too much, I panicked. Wasn't weight gain supposed to happen in the second trimester? If I wasn't gaining enough, I panicked. Was my baby all right?

In the second trimester the weight really began to pile on. I felt fat. Was I eating too much? I still didn't look pregnant. Was I eating too little?

In the third trimester I was constantly hungry. I ate what I wanted, when I wanted. I felt voluptuous. I felt obese too.

My doctor said I was "all baby." I knew that after delivery I would be a few pounds overweight, but I was convinced there was nothing diet and exercise wouldn't fix in a few weeks. I'd get my old body back in no time. How wrong I was. I was soon to learn that, not only was childbirth a completely life-changing experience, it was a completely body-changing experience as well.

When our beautiful baby boy was born I was exhilarated. I was also extremely fatigued. I looked at my thighs and stomach for the first time. If anything was going to trigger postpartum depression for me, this would. I still felt and looked pregnant.

In the days, weeks, and months that followed I never expected to feel so out of control as far as weight management was concerned. Some days I'd move the scales around on the floor trying to find the exact spot that gave the most favorable reading. It didn't work. There was no escaping the fact that at several months postpartum I was still a good twelve pounds over my prepregnancy weight.

Victoria Principal, the glamorous star of the TV series *Dallas,* once told *Redbook* magazine that it would not be in her "best physical interests to have a baby, so I've made the decision not to have any."

There are even reports of famous models and celebrities who are willing to pay women to carry their babies for them so that they won't have to put on any weight.

Early in my pregnancy a colleague at work asked why I wanted to ruin my body.

Is it true, then? Does having a baby ruin your figure?

Not according to some moms. They swear that having a baby actually improved their bodies. They got curves in the right places. It made them look more feminine.

But these women tended to be really thin, even boyish looking, before they got pregnant. They "needed" a few extra curves and a few extra pounds. The great majority of us, however, don't want any more curves! What we may worry about is the added fat gained during pregnancy. To have a baby you must increase your body fat by a certain amount. You can limit the amount you gain, of course, but you may as well resign yourself to seeing not just a swelling belly, but at least five to ten pounds of fat going onto your hips, thighs, and buttocks. The average gain in fat is just over eight pounds.

Most of us would agree that if the price for bringing a new life into the world is a changed body, we'll pay it. Having a baby is one of life's most wonderful and miraculous achievements. But this doesn't stop us wanting our figures back. Even the most contented mother-to-be might feel her contentment falter as she steps on the scales or catches a glimpse of her expanding silhouette. When baby is born this conflict and confusion doesn't go away. On the one hand you are ecstatic. Holding your sweet-smelling baby in your arms is perhaps the closest thing to bliss you have ever known. On the other hand, when you leave baby heaven and return to earth, you might feel unhappy about how out of shape you look.

Almost every new mom will find at some time or another that her desire to be a mother conflicts with social pressure to be thin. We don't need to search long for an explanation as to why we have this conflict.

It is during pregnancy and postpartum more than any other time in our lives that the cultural ideal of thinness is in direct contrast to the biology of being a woman.

If you, like me, have spent a lifetime watching your weight, the natural weight gain of pregnancy can cause anxiety. A professional dancer for many years, I had an even more significant reason to watch my weight. Up until a few years ago it was hard to find information and advice on how to cope with the bodily changes of pregnancy and weight loss postpartum. Books on pregnancy and childbirth focused almost exclusively on the health and care of baby. Seriously neglected were the health and well-being of mom. Thankfully, there are signs that this is beginning to change. There are now books, magazines, Web sites, and videos readily available that focus on getting back in shape and rebuilding your life after baby. The advice given is often intelligent, insightful, and informative. It is very positive that so many experts are beginning to recognize that mom's health and well-being is as important as the health and well-being of her children.

However, the subject of weight management during and after pregnancy was never covered in enough detail for me, or in a way I felt I could relate to. Sure, I wanted to read about the recommended weight gain during pregnancy and sensible diet and exercise during and after pregnancy, but there was so much more I wanted to know.

What about the underlying emotional issues involved? A woman's body is central to her definition of self. Just how do the bodily changes of pregnancy and postpartum really make us feel? I wanted to read other women's stories. How much did they eat? How much did they weigh? Did they exercise? How did they feel about their changing bodies? How did weight gain affect their lives? Why do some women gain more than others when pregnant? Why do some women snap back into shape after baby? How do they do it? Why do some of us never lose the extra pounds we gain with each new baby? How do partners feel about our changing bodies? What about women with eating disorders or postpartum depression—how does weight gain affect them?

Pregnancy Weight Management is for every woman who is concerned about weight management during and after pregnancy. Whether you are thinking of a having a baby, whether you are pregnant, or the mother of a two-week-old, a six-week-old, a five-month-old, or a toddler, this book will be of interest to you.

Part One looks at pregnancy weight gain and the impact this has on your life trimester by trimester. You will learn what a healthy weight gain is and can decide for yourself about "eating for two." Is it really necessary, or is it the cause of many postpartum weight problems? Also discussed will be the much-neglected issue of pregnant women who have eating disorders and how pregnancy weight gain affects them.

Part Two gives recommendations for weight management during pregnancy so that you can maximize your chances of a healthy, happy pregnancy.

In Part Three you will learn the truth about weight loss in the postpartum period. What happens to your body after delivery, what you will lose in the first week, what to realistically expect in terms of weight loss in the weeks and months and years that follow, and how big a factor weight gain is in postpartum depression will all be discussed.

Part Four looks at what partners think about your changing body. How weight gain can affect your sex life. Some of the information here may surprise you. You'll learn that partners can have weight management problems, too, during and after pregnancy. So next time you're feeling sorry for yourself, spare a thought for your partner. His or her life is being turned upside-down as well.

Part Five focuses on feeling good about yourself and your body after baby. Many questions concerning weight management are answered: Why is it so hard to lose the weight postpartum? Why am I not losing weight when my friend, who just had a baby, too, is? Is it harder to lose the weight the older you get? Will breastfeeding help me lose weight? What's my metabolic rate got to do with my weight? Is it true that certain foods can actually help me lose weight postpartum? When is it safe to exercise postpartum? How much exercise should I be doing to lose weight?

Diet and exercise recommendations are included to ensure optimum nutrition and health during and after pregnancy. But you won't see endless photographs of women who barely look pregnant or perfect-looking moms performing kegels with baby smiling in the background. You won't be given endless menus and diet plans that seem impossible to follow. Such "shape up" schemes to "bounce back after baby" are designed to get you motivated and are full of good intentions. But more often than not they make you feel even more despondent, when despite every effort you can't achieve the desired results. These programs don't always work because they fail to recognize that every one of us is unique. There is no diet or exercise plan that is going to work for every woman.

Pregnancy Weight Management will help you learn about your body and what works best for you, so you can make the right diet and exercise choices and design a weight management schedule that works for you and only you. The secret lies in trusting your body to know what it should weigh and recognizing how unique your body is. Only when I finally understood how wise and unique my body was did weight management become a success for me.

I also hope this book will help you understand, as I eventually did, that becoming a mother can offer a wonderful opportunity to finally liberate yourself from the diet mindset, which determines whether you have a good or bad day according to how much you weigh. It will show you that feeling healthy, energetic, and happy is far more important than the number you read on the scales.

Finally, there is one body basic every woman who has had a baby and is concerned about her weight should know:

Trying to get your "old body" back is impossible.

Before you throw up your hands in despair, let me point out that this is not as depressing as it sounds. It does not mean that you won't be able to lose weight. It does not mean that you will look heavy with child for the rest of your life. It does not mean that you won't ever have shape or form again—countless women have shown that weight management after pregnancy is not an impossible dream. It simply means that your old body does not exist any more. You have had a baby. Your body has changed forever. You have to learn about it all over again. You are entering a completely new stage in your life where the old rules don't apply anymore.

Baby has changed everything, including your body. And, if you have patience and motivation, and treat your body with the respect it deserves, you will find that this change is for the better.

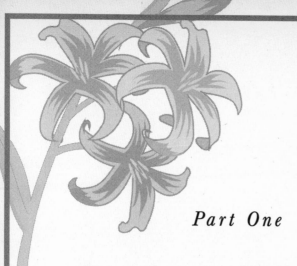

Part One

Looking Pregnant
Feeling Fat

The more pregnant I get the more
strangers smile at me. Why?
'Cause you're fatter than they are.
—A NON

In the Beginning

IF YOU ARE READING THIS BOOK, YOU ARE PROBABLY A WOMAN WHO watches her weight. You might be pregnant, a mother already, or planning to become pregnant. This is terrific. Weight management before, during, and after pregnancy is important for a healthy and happy transition to motherhood. Let's begin with prepregnancy weight management.

Here's what some new moms said about their weight before pregnancy:

> "I didn't plan for this pregnancy. I'd just started a new diet and was determined to lose weight. I stopped dieting as soon as I found out."

> "If only I had weighed less when I got pregnant. It's going to be so hard for me to lose all this weight after the baby."

> "When I got pregnant I was the slimmest I have ever been. It took me a long time to lose weight. Now I'm going to put it all back on again."

> "I wasn't happy with my weight when I got pregnant. I'm even more unhappy with how I look now."

When you get pregnant, your body shape is going to change. You will put on weight. Your self-esteem may be affected. If you are planning to have a baby, there is a way you can minimize some of the anxiety caused by the inevitable weight gain, and that is by making sure you are at a healthy body weight before you get pregnant.

If you are already pregnant or a mom and your prepregnancy weight was not ideal, don't despair—this book will show you how to get back on track. The point being made here is that a successful pregnancy and getting back in shape after baby just tend to be easier if prior to conception you were already at a healthy body weight. Perhaps if you are planning any future pregnancies this is something to bear in mind.

A healthy prepregnancy weight not only makes weight management less of a problem during and after pregnancy, it makes getting pregnant easier, too. Our bodies need a certain amount of body fat to maintain the menstrual cycle and ultimately to support pregnancy and lactation. If you are too thin or too heavy for your build, this can interfere with your menstrual cycle and make conception harder to achieve. To get pregnant, you first have to attain a healthy weight for height ratio and an essential fat store.

There is, however, no specific amount of weight loss or gain, no fat percentage that will make every woman conceive....

"I conceived when my body fat percentage was 15 percent."

"I've been trying to get pregnant for two years now. I have irregular periods."

"I got pregnant when I lost 20 pounds."

"I got pregnant when I gained 15 pounds."

All of us react differently to weight fluctuations, but it is clear that being over- or underweight tends to affect your fertility. In the words of Dr. Douglas, reproductive endocrinologist and infertility specialist at the Medical Center in Plano, Texas, "Extremes of body weight prepregnancy will affect your fertility. If you are significantly over or underweight you may or may not have periods, you may or may not be ovulating, but you will have problems conceiving."

In our diet-obsessed culture, maintaining an essential amount of body fat might be difficult for some to accept. Others may find weight loss a struggle. Whatever the case, if you want to have a baby and you are too heavy or too thin for your build, you need to decide what your priorities are. Some kind of middle ground needs to be found where you can maintain a weight that you are comfortable with and that also gives you the greatest chance of getting pregnant and having a healthy baby.

Giving Yourself and Your Baby-to-Be the Best Possible Start

Your health and your baby's health during pregnancy will be affected by your prepregnancy weight and general health. How much you weigh, what you eat, and how much you exercise are all important. Try, if you can, to give both yourself and your baby-to-be the best possible start.

"The best way to begin a pregnancy is when you are in good physical health, eating a well balanced diet, and not under excessive stress." says Dr. Stavia Blunt. "Throughout pregnancy diet, weight gain, lifestyle and physical activity have additional effects on the outcome of pregnancy. Adverse conditions may have adverse effects on the duration of the pregnancy and the birth weight of the baby." (Dr. Stavia Blunt, *Shaping Up During and After Pregnancy*, Summersdale, 1998, p. 30)

Simple leaflets on getting fit for pregnancy are readily available from your doctor. You will notice that they all stress the importance of weight management through healthy diet and exercise.

A Healthy Diet

Some experts believe that what you eat prior to conceiving is even more important than what you eat during pregnancy. Although good nutrition during pregnancy is crucial, the egg is a product of your diet up to the point of fertilization. A healthy diet maximizes your chances of a healthy pregnancy.

A healthy diet is low in fat, particularly animal fat, sugar and salt, refined carbohydrates, and processed food. This means cutting down on meat and dairy products such as cheese and milk and substituting with fish and vegetable protein. Cook with oils such as olive oil rather than butter. Eat whole grain bread and pasta and brown rice rather than the white alternatives and have as much fresh fruit and vegetables as possible. Avoid processed foods—they contain additives and lack nutrients. Try to use honey instead of sugar and cut down on sweets. Oil should be "cold pressed" and margarine should be "nonhydro-genated" to preserve the types of fat essential to our health called "essential fatty acids." You will also need to eliminate alcohol, cigarettes, and too much caffeine from your diet. These can deplete your body of the nutrients it needs.

Important Prepregnancy Nutrients

Folic acid is now considered essential for women thinking about pregnancy, especially if diet is poor. Make sure you take a folic acid supplement of 0.4 milligrams every day. Folic acid deficiency is associated with neural tube defects in developing infants. As well as watching your folic acid, pay particular attention to your intake of iron and vitamin D, as the requirements for these nutrients dramatically increases when you get pregnant.

According to *The Prescription for Nutritional Healing* (James and Phyllis Balch, Avery Publishing, 1997, p. 344), a balanced diet is crucial for women trying to conceive. Study after study has shown that remarkable improvements in fertility can result when diet and weight is healthy. Certain vitamins and minerals are even thought to improve fertility:

Vitamin A found in eggs, butter, green fruit, and vegetables. Deficiency can cause damage to the ovaries. (Warning: Too much vitamin A can be toxic. Consult a qualified doctor or nutritionist.)

Vitamin B found in whole grains, seeds, nuts, yeast. Many women who take the contraceptive pill are deficient in vitamin B. B vitamins are important for maintaining the health of the hormonal system. It is best to take a B complex vitamin as the B vitamins work together.

Vitamin C found in raw fruits and vegetables. Vitamin C fights the effects of stress and aging.

Vitamin E found in cold-pressed oils, whole grains, and green leafy vegetables improves ovulation.

Iron found in dark green leafy vegetables, eggs, and fish. Low levels of iron are associated with infertility in women.

Manganese found in whole grains, nuts, and onions. Another vitamin affected by the contraceptive pill. Manganese is important for the embryo to implant in the womb.

Magnesium found in seafood, whole grains, and milk. Again depleted by the contraceptive pill. It helps B vitamins get absorbed.

Selenium found in herring, tuna, and broccoli. This strengthens the immune system and makes vaginal mucus more sperm friendly. It should be taken with vitamins A, C, and E to help absorption. (Warning: Toxic in large amounts.)

Zinc found in seafood, milk, and whole grains. Low levels in women associated with miscarriage, implantation problems, and eating disorders.

Important warning: Be careful when taking dietary supplements. Self-prescription can be dangerous since some nutrients, such as vitamin A or selenium, can be toxic if you take too much. Make sure you get expert advice from your doctor or a qualified nutritionist.

Exercise

Exercise is key for prepregnancy weight management. Some of us lead very active lives. We never stop and are always on the go. Some of us lead very quiet sedentary lives. We are the ones who really need to exercise. Most of us fall somewhere in between. Whatever your activity level, everyone can benefit from a regular exercise program, especially if pregnancy is your goal. You will be preparing your body for the extra demands pregnancy will place on it. According to Dr. Jacobs, obstetrician, gynecologist, and infertility specialist at the Plano Medical Center in Texas, "In my experience, it's no myth that fit women have easier labors. They cope with the stresses of pregnancy and birth better also."

Your exercise program should include aerobic activity such as running, walking, or cycling for at least 45 minutes three to five times a week. Try to build muscle strength as well as aerobic capacity and overall endurance. Ideally, you should blend running and aerobics with non-impact sports such as walking and weight resistance training. Overall body strength and conditioning prior to pregnancy is a big plus. Concentrate on your abdominal muscles, back muscles, posture, and bending and lifting. Strength in these areas will make the physical changes of pregnancy easier to cope with.

Your Weight

To check your body weight prepregnancy, take a look at the BMI chart in Figure 1. A BMI of less than 18 or 19 means that you may be too thin. A body weight that is too high (over 27) means that you may be too heavy.

Consult with Your Doctor

A healthy weight, diet, and lifestyle will maximize your chances of conception and a healthy pregnancy. If you can, it might also be wise to visit your health care provider before attempting to get pregnant. Review your diet and exercise program, and talk to your doctor about it to ensure that you really are giving yourself and your baby-to-be the best possible start. Should you get pregnant, make sure you continue to ask about weight management, diet, and exercise throughout your pregnancy. Don't make the mistake of thinking that you can forget about your weight when you are pregnant. Regular weigh-ins at your doctor's won't let you forget.

You may feel embarrassed to discuss your weight with your doctor. Many women are. How much we weigh can be a sensitive area for us. We don't want the doctor to think we are vain or self-absorbed when we should be thinking about the health of the baby-to-be. But remember—your doctor is there not only for your baby-to-be, but for you. If weight is a concern for you, talk about it. You need to feel comfortable with this person who is going to guide you through one of the most incredible adventures of your life.

Figure 1: Your BMI

Height	Weight												
4ft 10in	91	96	100	102	110	115	119	124	129	134	138	143	148
4ft 11in	94	99	104	109	114	119	124	128	133	138	143	148	153
5ft	97	102	107	112	118	123	128	133	138	143	148	153	158
5ft 1in	100	106	111	116	122	127	132	137	143	148	153	158	164
5ft 2in	104	109	115	120	126	131	136	142	147	153	158	164	169
5ft 3in	107	113	118	124	130	135	141	146	152	158	163	169	175
5ft 4in	110	116	122	128	134	140	145	151	157	163	169	174	180
5ft 5in	114	120	126	132	138	144	150	156	162	168	174	180	186
5ft 6in	118	124	130	136	142	148	155	161	167	173	179	186	192
5ft 7in	121	127	134	140	146	153	159	166	172	178	185	191	198
5ft 8in	125	131	138	144	151	158	164	171	177	184	190	197	203
5ft 9in	128	135	142	149	155	162	169	176	182	189	196	203	209
5ft 10in	132	139	146	153	160	167	174	181	188	195	202	209	216
5ft 11in	136	143	150	157	165	172	179	186	193	200	208	215	222
6ft	140	147	154	162	169	177	184	191	199	206	213	221	228
Your BMI	**19**	**20**	**21**	**22**	**23**	**24**	**25**	**26**	**27**	**28**	**29**	**30**	**31**
			OPTIMAL		WEIGHT					OVERWEIGHT			

BMI (body mass index) Rating

2

Fertility Symbols
Are Never Thin

YOU ARE EXPECTING A BABY.

You are probably thrilled. This is one of the most exciting and wonderful things that has ever happened to you. You are maybe also a little apprehensive.

In little less than nine months you will undergo nothing less than a transformation. You will be pregnant. Then you will be a mom. There is so much for you to discover about yourself on this exciting journey. But along with any change there are also challenges and obstacles. One of the biggest challenges and obstacles may be a changed body image.

> Our sense of self begins to change as our bodies change. There are new sensations, limitations, and opportunities for self awareness. Part of this emotional adjustment is body image. Our once familiar "self" encounters the pregnant "self" and for some women these images can create a conflict. (Joan Marie Butler, *Fit and Pregnant*, Acorn, 1996, p. 30)

Here's what some women said when asked about gaining weight during pregnancy:

> "I gained thirty-two pounds but dreaded every weigh-in at the doctor's. One month I found out I had gained ten pounds. I wanted to cry. I knew I wanted my baby, but I hated what was going on with my body."

"I was five foot four and 110 pounds when I got pregnant. I ran about thirty-five miles a week and weight trained. My doctor told me to gain more weight than the average woman because I was too thin. I thought he was telling me I had to become fat."

"I'm not sure about having babies. I just couldn't put my body through that. I don't want to get fat."

"For the very first time I've had women responding in a survey that they won't get pregnant because they don't want to gain weight," Ann Kearney-Cooke, Ph.D., Director of the Cincinnati Psychotherapy Institute, is quoted as saying in *Fit Pregnancy* (Winter, 1998, p. 150). Cooke relates this phenomenon to a culture that has an "out of control obsession with thinness" and concern with image rather than the development of the self.

Fear of looking fat when your body changes can make feelings of embarrassment or inhibition likely during pregnancy. It's not hard to understand why. Our society is obsessed with youthful, perpetually adolescent standards of beauty. Being tall, firm-breasted, young, and thin, very thin, is today's cultural ideal of beauty. Many of us object to it, and can't live up to it—and yet it lingers on.

The thin ideal has a powerful hold over women in our culture. To put things in perspective, it can be illuminating to do a little research about other standards of beauty. Thin is not and was not always the ideal. The men of the Matsingenka, a remote tribe in Peru, for instance, have a fixed standard of beauty very different from ours. Shown pictures of Western models, the men grimaced and announced that they must have diarrhea. They approved instead of women with no waists and layers of fat. Plumper women have the ideal shape.

In centuries past the cultural standard of beauty was plump, not thin. The so called "Venus de Willendorf" female body type dominated the imagination of the known world for 25,000 years, as archeological finds from Iceland to Mongolia confirm. "Femina steatopygia," the woman with excessive fat, especially in the buttocks, was admired in Rubens' day, when famine and disease still reigned. It resurfaced as recently as the late Victorian times, when the plump wives of the masters of the Industrial revolution, as pictured by Ingres, were a comforting support for their husbands.

In the twentieth century our ideal of beauty has changed dramatically. First there was the hourglass, but still buxom, beauty of Marilyn Monroe. Since then, writes Jacqueline Shannon, "The standard of beauty we are held to has gotten increasingly rigid and more impossible to achieve." (*The New Mother's Body Book*, Contemporary Books, 1994, p. 227)

Today, plump is out and thin is in. We are pelted with messages telling us to be thinner, fitter, more shapely. Next time you are in a bookstore, take a look at the shelves and shelves of diet books or the rows of women's magazines that have the words "diet," "slim down," or "lose weight" on the cover. Small wonder women are ten times more likely than men to have eating disorders, such as anorexia or bulimia. In fact, eating disorders may just be the extreme on a universal spectrum. In today's culture, "to be a woman," writes Mary Pipher, "is to have a body image problem. For women, harmful eating plans are becoming the norm." (*Hunger Pains*, Ballantine, 1995, p. 5)

Here are some alarming statistics gathered from popular women's magazines and news reports:

- Women overestimate their body size. We think we are fatter than we are.
- About 80 percent of us think we are overweight when only about 25 percent of us are.
- Most of us hate our thighs, bottom, and stomach.
- The average American woman is 145 pounds and 5 feet 4 inches tall, but we wish we were at least twenty-five pounds lighter and a couple of inches taller.
- Every day millions of women in the United States are on a diet. The diet industry is booming.
- Concern about body weight starts young. In high schools, girls are skipping lunch.
- Young women don't want to stop smoking because they think it will make them gain weight.
- The birth control pill is rejected for the same reason.
- When asked what they fear most, many girls think gaining weight is more terrible than getting cancer or the threat of nuclear war.

Where do you fit into a thin-obsessed culture when you get pregnant? Fertility symbols are rarely depicted as thin. How on earth are you supposed to gain twenty-five pounds or so without feeling repulsive, ugly, and fat? "Pregnancy can trigger our most loathsome feelings about our body," writes Jennifer Louden, "sending us into incessant bouts of asking 'How fat do I really look? Come on, be honest.'" (*The Pregnant Woman's Comfort Book*, Harper Collins, 1995, p. 57)

Feeling Fat

Apprehension about getting bigger is just one of the many challenging feelings pregnancy weight gain can trigger. Women face a whole range of emotions when their bodies start to change. You might feel out of control since your body is changing without your conscious direction. You could feel invaded by another life form, or guilty for not enjoying everything about the process, because after all—isn't having a baby supposed to be the most wonderful thing a woman can do? There could be confusion about identity, your new role as mom, or even the meaning of life itself.

All these uncomfortable feelings may be encountered when your body changes shape. Sometimes "feeling fat" is about far more than weight gain. It is about deeper emotional conflicts that a changed relationship with your body brings.

Rethinking Your Body Image

During pregnancy, the transformation your body goes through goes hand-in-hand with the transformation your life is going through. Don't be surprised if you feel conflict between your need to feel attractive and the needs of the baby-to-be. It is how you deal with this conflict that matters—and that determines how healthy and happy you feel during your pregnancy. You could respond negatively to the conflict and see pregnancy as a frustrating barrier to thinness, feeling anxious about every pound you gain. You could feel disheartened: you were finally winning the battle of the bulge and now you have to call a temporary truce. You could decide to eat far more than is healthy for you and baby and deal with body anxiety by turning to food for comfort.

Or you could respond positively and follow the advice offered in this book. You could try to adjust your mindset about weight and body image so that you can maximize your chances and your baby-to-be's chances of health.

Rethinking your body image will take time and effort, but it could be one of the most important things you ever do for yourself and your baby-to-be. If you can focus on the exciting prospect of having a baby in your life, if you can respect the wisdom of your body, if you can concentrate more on health and well-being and less on how much you weigh, you will feel stronger, more empowered, more womanly, more fulfilled, and more comfortable with your body image than ever before.

3

Your Pregnant Body

I WAS A TYPICAL FIRST-TIME MOM. I THOUGHT BEING PREGNANT JUST meant a swelling abdomen. I was soon to learn differently. Aside from the weight gain, every part of me felt different. My hair, my skin, my eyes, my legs, my knees, my toes, my whole body felt pregnant. I had to learn to move in a different way.

All of us experience pregnancy in our own unique way. Some of us will get backache, tender breasts, nausea, and swollen feet, and some of us won't. But all of us will experience at least a few bodily changes. Many of the common complaints (see Figure 2) associated with pregnancy, such as backache or fatigue, will be related to weight gain. But although weight gain is the most obvious change, bear in mind that there are other physical changes as well caused by factors such as increased blood volume, hormonal changes, and so on. Most of these changes and complaints are temporary, but they can be unsettling.

You may feel magnificent when you get pregnant. Full of energy, joy, and inner calm. Or you may find the physical changes really hard to come to terms with both emotionally and physically. Either way, the first huge adaptation you will have to make is actually facing the reality that you are pregnant. Don't be surprised if you feel kind of ambivalent about it all, whether the pregnancy was planned or not. This is just your way of coping. A mixture of emotions is normal.

"I've been slim all my life. Gaining weight is going to feel really odd."

"I have always been in control of my body. Now I'm pregnant I've lost that control."

FIGURE 2: YOUR PREGNANT BODY—COMMON PROBLEMS

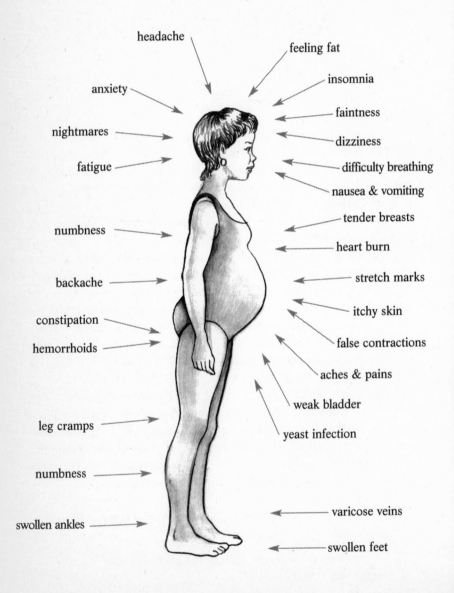

headache

feeling fat

anxiety

insomnia

nightmares

faintness

fatigue

dizziness

difficulty breathing

nausea & vomiting

numbness

tender breasts

heart burn

backache

stretch marks

constipation

itchy skin

hemorrhoids

false contractions

aches & pains

weak bladder

leg cramps

yeast infection

numbness

swollen ankles

varicose veins

swollen feet

"I'm not enjoying being pregnant as much as I thought I would."

"I'm going to have a baby. I don't see myself as a mom."

"I felt invaded when I was pregnant. There was this life inside me."

"I've never felt so feminine in my life. Being pregnant is wonderful."

"I'm eight months pregnant. I hate looking so huge."

At first you may just focus on the physical changes, so let's take a look at how your body changes during your pregnancy.

Remember that every pregnancy is different. What follows is just an approximation. Don't worry if you are a few weeks early or late for some of these changes. Or if you don't feel what you think you should feel. The best thing to do is check with your doctor if you are really concerned about your progress.

Pregnancy is usually dated from the first day of your last period, and this becomes week 1. Other books date conception as week 1. Conception usually occurs between one and three weeks after your period starts, so make sure you know what dating method you are using. As doctors tend to date from the day of your last period, this book will, too.

Your Changing Body in the First Trimester (The First Three Months—Weeks 1 to 14)

In the early weeks you may not even know you are pregnant. There might be some slight spotting which occurs when the embryo attaches itself to the wall of your womb, but you won't feel that different.

"I was really shocked when I found out I was pregnant. I was on the pill and I couldn't understand why I kept feeling so sick all the time. My breasts were also sore. I had to go up a cup size. My clothes felt tighter but I wasn't putting on weight. My mum thought I might be pregnant, but I didn't think it could be possible. I never forgot to take the pill. I did one of those home tests and I could not believe it when it went positive. I did another two tests just to make sure. I was shocked. I went to see

my doctor who confirmed that I was a good ten weeks pregnant." Jessica, age 29.

"I was disappointed in the early weeks. I really thought I
would feel pregnant. I kept doing home pregnancy tests to reassure myself that I really was going to have a baby. It wasn't until
week 12 that I really noticed a change." Sarah, age 37.

For most of us, breast enlargement and accompanying tenderness
are the first signs of pregnancy. At this early stage, surges of hormones
send blood and fluids to your breasts, stimulating the development of
milk-producing tissues and ducts. Over the course of your pregnancy
your breasts will grow one or two cup sizes and gain a pound or two of
tissue and fluids. You may notice more friction than usual from bras or
clothing. The areola, the pigmented circle around each nipple, enlarges
and darkens so that in about eight months it is ready to offer a good
target for a hungry baby. Montgomery glands, a ring of small bumps
on the areola that secrete an antibacterial substance, grow more prominent. Overall breast size increases as each week passes. Veins may
become more noticeable on the surface. Feelings of tenderness, heavi-
ness, and fullness are usual from week 5, but it's easy to miss this early
sign. Tender breasts are common before a period.

You probably won't start to feel pregnant until you are at least
ten to fourteen weeks pregnant. Around this time pregnancy hormones flood your system, and the volume of blood in your body
increases. By now your uterus has grown to the size of a small
orange, and your thyroid gland might look more prominent. You may
start feeling hot and sweaty. This is because your heart is pumping
extra blood. You won't really show in the first trimester, though,
especially if this is your first pregnancy. It isn't until approximately
the twelfth week that the uterus is too large to remain in your pelvis
and pushes out above the pubic bone.

By week 13 your baby-to-be is supported by the placenta and not
your hormones. The placenta weighs about an ounce now. It will weigh
on average about one and a half pounds at birth. You might notice a
small bump as the uterus moves up into your abdomen. Most women
breathe a sigh of relief around this time. The formation of the placenta
is an important transition for your baby-to-be to make, and once it has
occurred there is far less risk of miscarriage.

Although your weight shouldn't change much in these early months, your uterus is growing and your body is working incredibly hard to produce a baby. As well as breast tenderness, there are other early warning signs you might detect now. These include frequent urination, fatigue, headaches, and morning sickness.

Early in pregnancy as your uterus grows pressure is exerted on the bladder. You'll need to empty your bladder a lot, especially at night, throughout your pregnancy. Fatigue is another problem:

> "A few weeks after I found out I was pregnant the fatigue hit me. I would come home from work in the evening and have to lie down on the sofa. Most nights I was in bed by 8 o'clock. I did not wake refreshed from my sleep, though. I spent most of the night in the bathroom and every morning had the most terrible headache." Lucy, age 32

If you are used to having a lot of energy, first trimester fatigue may frustrate you. However much you sleep, you just feel tired and listless. Try to remember that the fatigue is due to the hormonal changes your body is going through as well as the metabolic demands of the fetus. You are doing nothing wrong. Energy tends to come back in the second trimester, but toward the end of your pregnancy fatigue returns again as you gain more weight. No one really knows why, but you may also suffer from headaches when you are pregnant—especially in this trimester.

Important note: Especially during the first trimester, don't take any medication of any kind without consulting your doctor first. Pain medications, such as Tylenol, that you took before could be dangerous for the fetus now.

Another early sign of pregnancy that is unmistakable is morning sickness.

> "I didn't feel pregnant until morning sickness struck. I woke up one morning and started vomiting. When the same thing happened the next day I knew I was pregnant." Anna, age 29

> "You forget how terrible morning sickness is. I do remember though that for a few months early in my pregnancy

it took over my life. It was as if my body was trying to rid itself of toxins. I couldn't bear the thought of food. Even toothpaste tasted foul. It really made me think about how casual my approach to food had been in the past. You have to think about every morsel you eat and live in fear of throwing up at any minute. I lost three pounds in the first trimester." Linda, age 37

Morning sickness is the sudden urge to throw up. It can strike at any time of the day and at any time in your pregnancy. You may be very lucky and not suffer from it at all, but for most women it is a classic trademark of the first few months. (Some experts think that pregnancy nausea may be nature's way of restricting calorie intake in the early months as relative malnutrition may encourage the placenta to grow and function better.) Certain foods or smells trigger nausea. For me it was the smell of burning wood! Nausea is caused by hormonal changes, a slowed digestion, and your growing uterus. It feels worse on an empty stomach. Morning sickness may stop you gaining any weight at all in the first trimester. Some women even lose weight, but generally if you are having a textbook pregnancy you should expect to be a few pounds heavier. But if you lose a few pounds or don't gain any at all, this is perfectly normal.

The reason weight gain should be minimal now is because your baby-to-be is still very tiny. At thirteen weeks he or she is only two or three inches long and weighs about half an ounce. As tiny as your baby-to-be is, though, remember that an incredible amount of development is taking place. Just seven days after the fertilized egg implants in your womb it becomes an embryo. Nerve development begins around week 4 and the heart starts to beat. Between weeks 9 and 13 the baby-to-be starts to look more human. Ears and eyes form and the face begins to take shape.

If you are concerned about looking fat when you are pregnant, understanding exactly what is happening to your body and why will help you come to terms with the weight gain. Buying a pregnancy calendar or a book that outlines how your baby-to-be develops and grows in detail will make it clear to you that there is a reason for every pound you gain. Bear in mind that every pregnancy is different and no baby will develop in exactly the same way. Don't worry if you are a few weeks ahead or behind in development.

The Second Trimester
(Months 3 to 6—Weeks 14 to 24)

During the first trimester, if you don't feel too tired, apprehensive, irritable, and nauseated, you can enjoy being pregnant without actually looking pregnant. But during the second trimester, your body will start to change as you gain weight.

> "Now I really got hungry. It was wonderful to be able to eat again after months of gagging at the thought of food. After gaining no weight in the first trimester my weight shot up twenty pounds to 150 pounds. It was strange to feel so large. I have always felt in control of my weight and now I lost that control." Jessica, age 29

> "Just can't believe I'm pregnant. I'm so happy. I've always wanted a baby of my own. I'm five foot eight and was about 128 pounds when I got pregnant. I'm 142 pounds now. I get frustrated sometimes 'cause no one is interested in me anymore. They only ask about my baby. Nobody seems to look me in the eye anymore either. They just stare at my stomach. I hate it when they tap it. My girlfriends tell me I'm blooming. I think I look huge." Penny, age 29

During the second trimester bodily change will be impossible to ignore. Weight gain is rapid. Clothes start getting too tight as your uterus expands. Extra weight and fluids will also show up in a filled-out face. Even your nose may feel bigger as nasal tissues may swell— nasal tissues swell because pregnancy hormones in the blood increase blood flow to the nose's mucous membranes that soften and swell in response—one reason why pregnant women are often prone to stuffy noses or nose bleeds. Your breasts will seem more sensitive, and as they enlarge stretch marks may appear on the skin. You may get sweaty as your metabolism works overtime to keep you and your baby-to-be nourished. Some women notice a deepening of skin pigmentation in certain areas. Pigmented areas such as freckles, the nipples, and areolas may become darker and more prominent, especially when exposed to sunlight. Usually this fades after the baby is born. There could be a dark line down the center of your abdomen. You may get tiny dilated blood vessels on your arms, face, and legs. These little red squiggles that suddenly appear underneath your skin are due to increased blood volume as well as the hormonal changes of pregnancy.

By week 16 your uterus is about the size of a large grapefruit. Your bump might start to show now. By week 20 your waistline will have probably gone and your navel will flatten out. Week 20 is half way through your pregnancy. As early as now you could find out the sex of your baby-to-be. You should also feel some movements. By week 22 the top of your uterus will be parallel with your belly button.

Not surprisingly, weight gain brings with it an assortment of discomforts as your body adapts. Leg cramps, insomnia, swollen ankles, heartburn, backache, aches and pains, numbness in the arms and legs, and constipation are common at this time.

Late in this trimester and throughout the third, many women notice that they get violent cramps in their legs, especially in the middle of the night. These pains are caused by muscle spasms. You could also get pain radiating from your hip down to your leg. This pain is called sciatica, and it is caused by the uterus putting pressure on the sciatic nerve. It's also quite usual to get some pain in your belly or pelvis in mid-pregnancy. As your uterus grows into your abdomen, it stretches the supporting ligaments. You could also suffer from numb arms and legs. This is because your belly is putting pressure on sensitive nerves, causing numbness and tingling.

Your expanding belly might make finding a comfortable sleeping position hard. You can't sleep on your stomach any more, and sleeping on your back is not recommended by your doctor.

Another unpleasant side effect of pregnancy weight gain can be swelling. Blood and plasma volume increase dramatically in the second half of pregnancy—by as much as eight pounds. You need this extra blood to nourish your baby-to-be. Your growing uterus puts pressure on the blood vessels that return fluid from the legs. Feet and ankles may start swelling as your weight increases. If you have swollen ankles and feet, you may find you get swollen hands and fingers too.

Extra weight and a growing uterus alter your center of gravity, making back pain more likely. Lower back pain occurs in most pregnancies. Women often draw their shoulders back and sway their backs to compensate as they walk. This curvature of the lower back is what causes the strain. The stronger the abdominal muscles are before pregnancy, the less likely you are to get back strain.

Some women experience heartburn in this trimester and in the third as well. Again this is associated with an increase in weight. The regurgitation of gastric contents is caused by the compression of your stomach by your expanding uterus and by the relaxation of the cardiac sphincter muscle which lies between the stomach and the esophagus. The cardiac sphincter relaxes because of high levels of progesterone and other hormones, not because your baby-to-be's hair is tickling your windpipe. Later on in your pregnancy the uterus will press more and more on your stomach, and acid may rise from the stomach into your windpipe giving you a nasty burning sensation.

As your weight increases, you could be prone to bouts of constipation, which will make you feel even heavier. The hormones progesterone and estrogen relax muscles involved in digestion and slow the digestive process when you are pregnant. Bloating, indigestion, constipation, and, worse still, hemorrhoids are likely as the growing uterus tends to compress your bowels.

Toward the end of this trimester, you might feel as if everything is getting bigger except your bladder and your brain! Urination will be even more frequent. You may also start getting a little forgetful and disorganized, probably because you have a lot on your mind. Studies have shown that during a woman's pregnancy her brain does actually shrink (at least something is shrinking!), but this is only temporary. Besides, brain size has nothing to do with intelligence.

It isn't all bad news, though. There are a few positive changes now to offset the discomforts. The glow your skin gets, for instance, due to the increased blood flow of pregnancy. Acne, if you have it, tends to improve during pregnancy as pregnancy suppresses the production of androgens, a common cause of acne. The downside is that some moms-to-be may suddenly react to hormonal changes with a breakout of pimples. If this happens, certain medications that are high in vitamin A, such as Accutane, should be avoided. Another pregnancy bonus is thicker hair. At any time about 90 percent of your hair is in a growing phase. The remaining 10 percent has stopped growing and is in a resting phase where new hair forms. After a few months of resting, the old hair is shed and the new one grows. During pregnancy hormonal shifts can slow the shift from growing to resting and fewer hairs are shed. You should have thicker hair. Less appealing is the tendency to grow facial hair, which also happens during pregnancy. You might find that your hair gets oilier, or in some cases dryer. Don't be surprised if your nails grow more quickly, too.

Some women find during the second trimester that their libido increases. If you can find the energy, the second trimester is the best time to have sex. Fatigue and morning sickness in the first trimester are inhibiting, and in the third trimester finding a position that will not crush your partner or cause you discomfort will be a challenge.

The third trimester is a period of rapid growth for your baby-to-be and therefore a period of significant weight gain. By week 20 your baby-to-be could be about 11 inches long and weigh around 15 ounces. At week 21, the baby-to-be starts to gain fat, and ears and eyelids are well formed. At week 22, he or she begins to sleep and wake. You could hear a heartbeat. Genitals will be distinct.

At week 23, growth slows down, but she develops in other ways. The first momentous sensation of movement can occur anytime between the fourteenth and twenty-sixth week. The average is between the eighteenth and twenty-second week. A slender woman may notice movements earlier than an overweight woman. Second-time moms also often notice them earlier than first-time moms. It's impossible to describe how the movements feel. You might even mistake them for hunger pains or gas. As your pregnancy progresses, though, they become stronger and easier to recognize. More than seeing the ultrasound or hearing the heartbeat or gaining weight, feeling your baby-to-be move can make a pregnancy seem more real.

As this trimester draws to a close you will lose your waistline, clothes won't fit, and you will be noticeably heavier. But weight gain, lack of coordination, bleeding gums, constipation, backache, yeast infections, swollen ankles, and the constant need to urinate are offset by glowing skin, shining hair, and the miracle of feeling new life inside you.

The Third Trimester
(the Last Three Months—Weeks 24 to 40)

"I must have gained close to forty pounds by now. I just feel like I have been this huge forever. My body doesn't feel like it belongs to me anymore." Lucy, age 29, is in her thirty-ninth week.

"I think my body looks disgusting. I don't like being so heavy and uncoordinated." Gloria, age 36, is in her thirty-fourth week.

"The physical changes alarm me. I had a slim athletic build—five feet seven and a 125 pounds. I've now transformed into a rounder shape and gained about thirty pounds. I've watched my abdomen swell, my hips swell, my bottom swell. Everything swells. I feel so pregnant, from my face right down to my toes." Debra, age 31, is in her fortieth week.

"When my belly started to expand I would look in the mirror and see this person I didn't recognize. This wasn't my body. This wasn't how I looked. For a while I really didn't know who I was anymore." Linda, age 33, is in her fortieth week.

For most of the third trimester you will continue to gain weight rapidly. Between weeks 24 to 31, your uterus grows to the size of a football. Fluid retention could make your face look puffy. The top of your uterus is now between your belly button and your rib cage and your stomach feels squashed. You'll have to eat smaller and smaller amounts as your pregnancy progresses. You'll feel strong movements from the baby-to-be as he kicks his arms and legs. Your breasts could feel large and uncomfortable. Around week 28, breasts may start leaking colostrum, which is a prelude to the milk you will give your baby if you opt to nurse. Around twenty-nine weeks your heart is working really hard and blood volume increases dramatically. You will feel even more pressure up against your stomach, liver, diaphragm, and intestine. By thirty weeks your uterus will be well above your belly button.

In the last ten weeks, as your baby nears birth weight, it's common to feel pressure or pain in your hips. Most of the weight gain now will be not just on your belly, but in your hips, bottom, and thighs. We typically put on weight there anyway, but during pregnancy we need these extra fat stores for breastfeeding after baby is born.

As you get nearer to your due date, your belly should contain about seven pounds of baby and several pounds of placenta, uterus, and fluid. Don't be surprised that carrying all this extra weight throws you off balance. Your center of gravity changes as the fetus grows out of your pelvis and tips forward into your abdominal muscles. Your body is also releasing the hormone that prepares you for childbirth, and this relaxes your hip and knee joints making you more prone to falls. Extra weight will make you less light on your feet and also a little uncoordinated.

At thirty-three weeks, weight gain should be faster than ever in your pregnancy. This should continue to about thirty-six weeks when blood volume has increased by 40 percent. At thirty-four weeks the baby-to-be may drop down and you may notice a change in your abdomen shape.

You may sometimes feel as if your belly has become the main attraction wherever you go! The size and growth rate of your uterus indicates whether the fetus is developing on track. That's why your doctor measures your stomach from week 20 onwards. Your uterus grows about a centimeter each week, so this external measurement from your pubic bone to the top of your uterus should approximately equal your week of pregnancy. For example, your belly may measure about 22 centimeters at twenty-two weeks, but this proportion isn't always exact. If your measurement is too small or too large, your doctor will check with an ultrasound scan.

At thirty-seven weeks, weight gain should slow down or stop. You could find breathing easier but you will still need to visit the restroom a lot. At thirty-eight weeks you are not likely to gain much more weight. You could notice a strange sensation inside your vagina as baby pushes down against your pelvic floor muscles.

In the final weeks when weight gain stabilizes, your cervix should begin to soften in preparation for birth, which could happen anytime between weeks 38 and 42. Very few babies are born on the due date their doctors give them, although about 75 percent are born within ten or so days of it.

Weight gain in the final trimester can make you feel quite uncomfortable and tired. You may find that the extra weight makes you prone to itchy skin eruptions too. This is called prickly heat, an itchy red rash, that usually appears in the skin and blocks the escape of perspiration from the sweat glands. Chafing may occur in skin folds, such as under the breasts. Very dry abdominal skin can get irritated, too.

The extra weight may also make you feel out of breath or even dizzy if you stand or sit for too long in one place or if you don't eat enough. If you lie on your back the blood supply to your baby and to you is limited as the uterus compresses arteries, and you will feel faint.

You might get sore ribs as well. This is caused by the top of your uterus pressing on your ribs. You might get odd aches and pains around your abdomen and sides. This is called round ligament pain and it usually strikes from the sixth month. It is caused by hormonal changes and an increased blood supply and added weight stressing your ligaments. You might also notice brief, shooting pains in your vagina caused by pressure on the nerves.

Varicose veins are a common problem for pregnant women. They tend to run in families. If your mother suffered from them, you may. Rapid weight gain contributes to the problem as your growing uterus presses against the veins in your pelvis and slows the return flow of blood from your legs to your heart. Sluggish circulation can aggravate or bring on enlarged veins in your legs. These might ache some days, especially after you've been standing. In Chapter 10, we'll see how you can alleviate the various pregnancy weight related discomforts.

If you feel very uncomfortable in the final trimester, it can be helpful to know that during this trimester your baby-to-be is making incredible advances. There is an explanation for every pound you have gained.

At twenty-four weeks she may have a sense of touch. She could be able to hear and may respond to music and sounds outside the womb. She could even recognize your voice. At twenty-six weeks, eyelids could open for the first time. Some light gets in through your abdominal wall and brightens her shadowy world. At twenty-seven weeks, your baby-to-be can move freely in your womb. At twenty-eight weeks, she could be around 14 inches long and weigh a couple of pounds. Heartbeat is about 120–140 beats a minute, double what yours is. At twenty-nine to thirty-one weeks your baby-to-be could hear both your voice and your partner's and her taste buds might be developed. Between weeks 32 and 34, if she is in a breech position—head up—she should turn head down, although 4 percent of babies stay head up and are born that way. Her eyes may now open for some time and she could start learning to focus. She usually has fingernails, and her lungs are getting ready for breathing on their own. At thirty-four weeks she might be around 17 inches long and weigh about 5 pounds. At thirty-five weeks, you can probably feel parts of your baby-to-be through your tummy. At thirty-six weeks she could weigh about 6 pounds and be about 18 inches long. Her head could engage (descend into the pelvis) at thirty-seven weeks. At thirty-eight weeks your baby-to-be will have grown a few more inches and gained a few more pounds. She is ready to make you a mom!

As your pregnancy draws to a close, you will probably feel enormous, exhausted, and apprehensive, but there will probably be excitement and anticipation for delivery day as well. The day when your baby-to-be finally arrives. The day when your body becomes your own again, and you hope some semblance of normality will return.

4

What's a Healthy Weight Gain During Pregnancy

THE QUESTION MANY PREGNANT WOMEN WANT TO ASK EACH OTHER IS, how much weight have you gained? Unfortunately, though, comparing oneself with others can often be a little unsettling.

One woman gains fifteen pounds in the first two months, another loses a few pounds in the first month, another in her third trimester has gained fifty pounds, and another gains only twenty throughout her pregnancy.

Just what is right? How much is a healthy weight gain?

Weight Gain During Pregnancy

If you were wealthy and born in the 1800s, you were probably plump and proud of it. Should you have gotten pregnant, you would have spent much of your time in "confinement." Pregnancy was considered a "delicate" condition. You were expected to do very little. You probably ate a lot out of boredom. After all, you were "eating for two." You would have stayed at home and avoided travel. You would have been huge by the time you delivered.

As the century drew to a close there were signs that the days of "porking up" during pregnancy were over. Consider this advice given to pregnant women in 1883 (Wilhelmine D. Schott, *Health Hints to Women*, New York: Charles P. Somerby, 1883, p. 87)

> Eat only twice daily....Excessive indulgence in food has
> hurried more people to the grave than war, famine, pestilence
> and alcohol combined...its ravages are ceaseless; from year to

year it pursues its work of destruction without pause or inter-
ruption...it spreads disease and death amongst all classes, ages,
sexes and conditions—maidens and matrons—infants and
children—the feeble and robust—all are swept indiscriminately
into the grave by this fell destroyer.

The tide turned fully in the 1950s when doctors were advising
pregnant women not to gain more than ten or fifteen pounds. It was
thought that this would mean a smaller baby and an easier birth. Fat
during pregnancy was considered unfit and unhealthy. Aren't you glad
you weren't pregnant then?

So what is considered ideal for the pregnant woman today?
What's the healthy weight gain recommended by doctors?

The committee on Nutritional Status During Pregnancy recom-
mends a weight gain of twenty-five to thirty-five pounds. It seems that
doctors have gone for the happy medium. Research has shown that
gaining too little or too much is dangerous for you and baby-to-be.

Gaining Too Much

"I was five foot nine, 135 pounds before I got pregnant.
I've gained nearly forty-five pounds with this baby. I did not
think I would gain so much. I'm a fitness instructor and I
should know better. But like a lot of first-time moms I saw this
pregnancy as a time to really relax and enjoy. I snacked when
I wanted. Every day I ate chocolate and cookies before I went
to bed. In the first trimester the food helped me fight the
nausea, and now with just a few weeks to go it gives me
energy. I get so tired." Martha, age 35, in her third trimester

If you start gaining too much weight, you may find that your
doctor makes no mention of your weight gain unless your health and
your baby-to-be's health is seriously at risk. Your doctor may believe
that the weight you gain over and above what your baby-to-be needs
is up to you. But, throwing caution to the wind and eating all you
want when you are pregnant is not a good idea. When you gain too

much weight, you are not doing either yourself or your baby-to-be any favors.

You are more liable to get backache from overworking your back muscles. Fatigue will become a way of life. Your doctor will find it hard to measure your belly, and you are at increased risk of heart disease, hypertension, gestational diabetes, and respiratory problems. When it comes to delivery, the baby may become so large that a vaginal delivery will be difficult, and if you have a cesarean the excess fat will make surgery difficult. Postoperative problems are more likely, too.

As well as putting your own health at risk, you risk the health of your baby-to-be. If you overindulge in junk food, fat, and sugar, your baby-to-be won't be getting the nutrients she needs. You also increase the chances of your baby-to-be getting spina bifida and other neural tube defects. According to some researchers, you also increase a daughter's risk of getting breast cancer.

Before you reach for that second helping of ice cream, remind yourself that the more weight you gain in pregnancy the harder it will be to lose weight postpartum. Excessive weight gain stretches your skin and you could get permanent stretch marks. Postpartum sagging in the breasts is more likely, too. The larger your baby, the more trauma to the pelvic region. And finally, the more weight you gain, the lower your self-esteem.

Gaining Too Little

"I really don't want to gain much with this pregnancy. I'm going to be careful and not overeat. I've always been good at controlling my appetite. So far I've only gained fourteen pounds and I'm nearing the end of the second trimester. I want to keep my weight gain under twenty pounds if I can. Nobody can believe I'm nearly six months pregnant. I feel really proud of myself." Cathryn, age 29, in her second trimester

If you have always been able to diet successfully and keep your weight low, it might be tempting during pregnancy to try and do the same. You restrict your food intake and exercise a lot. You feel okay, so your baby-to-be must be okay. And even if you feel a little weak, it doesn't matter—baby-to-be will take what he needs from you. He won't be harmed.

Unfortunately, it doesn't work that way. Women who gain less than twenty pounds and who were not overweight before they got pregnant are playing a dangerous game. Don't think that your baby-to-be is getting what he needs from your fat stores. He isn't. "Pregnancy is never a time for weight loss or maintenance, because a fetus can't survive on a mother's fat stores alone since they provide calories but no nutrients." (Eisenberg, Murkhoff, and Hathaway, *What to Expect When You're Expecting*, Workman, 1996, p. 148)

Initially, if you diet when pregnant the fetus tends to draw on maternal fat stores, but the extent to which this occurs is not certain. Once the mother's weight falls below a critical threshold, or when diet is severely restricted, fetal health is at risk. At this point diet restriction will affect the baby-to-be as well as you. Inadequate diet is especially harmful during the third trimester when fetal growth is most rapid.

Babies whose mothers gain under twenty pounds are more likely to be premature, and they are usually small for their gestational age. Babies born under six pounds have a higher rate of stillbirth, poor development, mental retardation, and lowered intelligence. Inadequate nutrition is associated with an increased risk of growth problems or fetal restriction. Inadequate weight gain is associated with neurological problems, learning disabilities, and even cerebral palsy. Also, women who diet during pregnancy may find that they can't breastfeed their babies successfully because there are insufficient fat stores to draw on to produce milk.

Why You Should Gain Twenty-Five to Thirty-Five Pounds

"Babies who have a birth weight of between six and eight pounds just do better," says Dr. Jacobs. Doctors recommend a weight gain in the region of twenty-five to thirty-five pounds because this produces the healthiest babies, weighing around six to eight pounds.

Let's break down how you will gain weight to show why you need to gain about twenty-five pounds minimum. A twenty-five to thirty-five pound weight gain allows six to eight pounds for baby-to-be and fourteen to twenty-four pounds for placenta, breasts, additional blood and fluid, and other by-products.

Imagine you had a total weight gain of thirty-one pounds during your pregnancy. Your weight gain would break down in approximately this way:

Baby—8 pounds
Amniotic fluid—2 pounds
Uterus expansion—2 pounds
Maternal breast tissue—2 pounds
Body fluid—4 pounds
Blood volume—4 pounds
Placenta—2 pounds
Fat and protein stores—7 pounds
Total average—31 pounds overall weight gain.

The growing baby-to-be and its needs account for about twenty-four pounds in this scenario. About this twenty-four pounds you have little choice. About the deposit of fats and fluids within you, which should amount to between five and ten pounds, you have a little more choice, but it is important to choose to put on those extra pounds.

Why do you need an extra five to ten pounds of fat in your own body?

Five to ten pounds over and above what the baby needs is thought to improve your chances of delivering a healthy, normal baby. Here's why:

During the first trimester the weight you gain prepares your body for the needs of the growing fetus.

In the second trimester the weight you gain is added to your own fat stores. You suddenly start getting fuller in the breasts, abdomen, hips, and thighs. This second trimester weight gain is vital because during the third trimester when your baby is growing fast, your metabolic rate changes. It is the weight stored during the second trimester that now nourishes your body, while the calories you consume go to your baby-to-be. You will also need a few extra pounds for breast-feeding later.

In short, each day of the whole nine months is crucial for your baby's development. He needs a constant supply of nutrients. He can't get all that he needs from your fat stores at any time in your pregnancy.

Your baby-to-be needs you to be well nourished. If you are not, he will suffer.

This is so important I'll emphasize it again: *Never, ever try to restrict your weight gain beyond what is recommended by your doctor.*

Other Factors Influencing Pregnancy Weight Gain

Sometimes the twenty-five to thirty-five pound rule won't apply. There are a number of other factors that can influence pregnancy weight gain.

How much weight is right for you to gain depends, first of all, on how much you weighed before coming pregnant. If you were twenty or thirty pounds overweight, you probably will need to gain less. Dr. Jacobs observes that some overweight patients don't gain much weight at all. On the other hand, women who were underweight before becoming pregnant will need to gain more than twenty-five to thirty-five pounds.

According to some experts there should be no general recommendation for weight gain during pregnancy ". . . as the ideal weight gain will vary according to the mother's pre-pregnancy weight." (Dr. Stavia Blunt, *Shaping Up During and After Pregnancy*, Summersdale, 1997, p. 43) Your prepregnancy weight is important when considering a healthy weight gain during pregnancy. How much weight you should gain will depend on how much you weighed before you got pregnant. There is a clear relationship between your prepregnancy weight, the weight gain during pregnancy, and your baby's birth weight.

If you're not sure if you are under or overweight, Figure 3 might help. Do bear in mind, though, that this table is for a woman of medium build in her prepregnancy state. Your build may be very different and you will want to discuss this with your doctor. Figure 4 may also help and give you some idea of how much you should gain during pregnancy. According to the National Academy of Sciences Institute of Medicine a woman who is underweight should gain in the region of twenty-eight to forty pounds total. A woman of normal weight should gain twenty-five to thirty-five pounds, and an overweight woman should gain fifteen to twenty-five pounds. Women who are obese

FIGURE 3: HEIGHT TO WEIGHT CHART (MEDIUM FRAME)

HEIGHT (IN)	WEIGHT = NORMAL	UNDERWEIGHT	OVERWEIGHT	OBESE
57	102-133	101	134-150	151
58	104-136	103	137-153	154
59	107-140	106	141-157	158
60	108-142	107	143-159	160
61	111-145	110	146-164	165
62	114-149	113	150-168	169
63	116-152	115	153-172	173
64	119-156	118	157-176	177
65	122-160	121	161-180	181
66	124-163	123	164-184	185
67	127-167	126	168-188	189
68	130-170	129	171-192	193
69	133-174	132	175-196	197
70	135-178	134	179-200	201

Source: Metropolitan Life Height and Weight Tables

FIGURE 4: PREGNANCY WEIGHT GAIN CHART

HEIGHT	5FT	5FT 2IN	5FT 4IN	5FT 6IN	5FT 8IN	5FT 10IN
Underweight	<102lbs	<107lbs	<116lbs	<123lbs	<130lbs	<138lbs
Normal	102-132lbs	107-141lbs	116-152lbs	123-161lbs	130-171lbs	138-181lbs
Overweight	133-147lbs	142-157lbs	153-170lbs	162-180lbs	172-191lbs	182-202lbs
Obese	>148lbs	>158lbs	>171lbs	>181lbs	>192lbs	>203lbs

IF YOU ARE-	UNDERWEIGHT	NORMAL	OVERWEIGHT	OBESE
You should gain when you are pregnant	28-40lbs	25-35lbs	15-25lbs	15lbs

Source: National Academy of Sciences

should not try to lose weight, but should keep their pregnancy weight gain to fifteen pounds or less.

If you are underweight for your age and height, doctors recommend that you gain weight in the first trimester so that you start the second close to your ideal weight. Then you can aim to gain the required twenty-five to thirty-five pounds on top of that. A total weight gain of twenty-eight to forty pounds is advised.

If you are significantly overweight, you will probably be advised to gain less than twenty-five pounds, though never less than fifteen pounds and only on a very nutritious eating plan.

Pregnancy is never a time to diet. Remember, a fetus cannot survive on your fat stores alone. They provide calories, but not the nutrients your baby needs. Overweight women who gain less than fifteen pounds have infant mortality rates twice those of overweight women who have adequate weight gain.

If you are a teenager, a smoker, or have a low body fat percentage, you should aim for a weight gain at the upper end of the range, and if you are less than five feet two inches you should try to gain weight at the lower end of the range because of possible problems a large baby might bring when delivery time comes.

How much weight is right for you to gain can depend on your baby's birth weight. There is a good chance that a huge weight gain will deliver a big baby, but birth weight and maternal weight gain do not always correlate. A fifty-pound weight gain can yield a six- or seven-pound baby. A twenty-pound weight gain can yield an eight-pound baby.

Believe it or not, the largest newborn recorded weighed twenty-six pounds. Don't panic! It is extremely rare to deliver a baby larger than twelve or thirteen pounds. Your baby's birth weight may be determined by other factors. Your diet, for instance. If the weight was gained on junk food with little nutritional value, you can still deliver a small baby. Also, women with larger builds tend to have larger babies. Your own birth weight may be significant. If you were born small, your baby may tend to be small, too. The length of time you carried your baby is also important for birth weight. Certain diseases, pregnancy disorders, and the use of drugs can alter newborn weight, too.

Your doctor can give you some idea of how big your baby is going to be by palpating your abdomen, by measuring the top of your uterus, and by sonogram. He or she can make a guess, but sometimes the guesses are a pound or so off.

If your baby is large, it does not mean you will have a difficult delivery. The determining factor in delivery is not how large the baby is, but whether it can fit through your pelvis. If your doctor suspects this might be a problem, he or she will let you go into labor normally, and if problems occur give you a boost of oxytocin or recommend a cesarean.

> "I'm very short, but my partner is six feet two. I'm afraid
> my baby is going to be big and that I'll have a difficult labor."

It simply isn't true that large partners make large babies. And when it comes to childbirth, nothing is ever certain. How easy your labor is depends on your contractions and how mobile you are. Even the biggest babies can get through the smallest gaps.

It is also not true that the size of your baby shows up in how you are carrying. Figure 5 shows three women all carrying in different ways in the seventh month. A small woman carrying low and small may give birth to a nine-pound baby, and a woman with a bigger build who is carrying higher and wider may give birth to a six-pound baby. Sometimes women with tight abs carry higher than those with lax abdominal wall muscles, but again this is not always the case. There are so many variations. It all depends on your size, your build, and the baby's position and size. You may carry high, low, big, small, or wide. You will carry in your own unique way. No two pregnant women look alike. Your belly—high, low, pointy, or big all around—only predicts that you're having a baby. "How you carry has to do with your body type, how much room you have between your pelvis and diaphragm, and even how the baby is lying in the womb," says Mary P. O'Day, M.D., assistant professor of maternal and fetal medicine at Baylor College of Medicine, in Houston. (Quoted from *American Baby* article by Sarah McCraw Crow, Feb. 1999, p. 51)

How you are carrying won't affect your overall weight gain, either. But how you are carrying may make you appear heavier. Two women of similar build can gain the same amount of weight, but the one who

FIGURE 5: THREE OF THE MANY DIFFERENT WAYS A WOMAN CAN CARRY

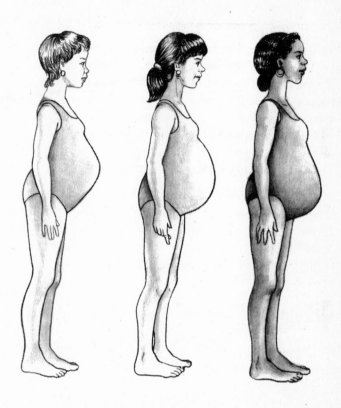

is carrying high and round, for instance, may appear heavier than the one who is carrying small and low.

So what if you are carrying twins? Should you gain twice as much? The answer is no. Although your weight gain will increase significantly, it will not be in the range of fifty to seventy pounds. Recommended weight gain in the case of twins is more in the range of thirty-five to forty-five pounds. Also, if you are carrying more fetuses you will be considered high-risk and your weight gain, exercise, and diet will be closely monitored by your doctor.

Pregnancy myth: Boys are all around. Girls are out in front.

How you carry depends entirely on you, your baby, and your body. You can't tell the sex of a baby by how you carry. Traditionally, first-time moms have neater bumps simply because their bodies haven't been pregnant before. Second and third pregnancies tend to spread out more. It's nothing to do with sex hormones affecting your shape.

Pregnancy myth: Small feet mean a difficult labor.

Amazingly, this might have some truth in it. Research has shown that the size of your feet gives some indication of the size of your pelvis. Usually a small pelvis is bad news, but not always. A small pelvis may not necessarily mean you will have a difficult birth. It depends on how big your baby is.

How Pregnancy Weight Should Be Gained

"I've put on twenty pounds already and I've just started my second trimester. Should I only gain another five pounds now?"

You should aim to keep your weight gain slow and steady. "The rate at which you gain is almost as important as how much you should gain. Slow steady weight gain during the whole pregnancy is ideal," says Connie Marshall, in her book *From Here to Maternity* (Conmar, 1997, p. 20)

Doctors recommend that during the first trimester you gain only three to four pounds. During the second trimester you should gain about a pound a week, or twelve to fourteen pounds in all. During the seventh and eighth months you should continue to gain about a pound a week. Finally, in the ninth month you should gain only a pound or two or even nothing at all, making a total gain of eight to ten pounds in the third trimester.

It is during the second and third trimester that you need to gain most of your weight. This is when the fetus is growing fast. Even if you have gained too much in the first trimester, you should not restrict your food intake now or diet. It could harm both you and your baby-to-be.

It's impossible to follow this weight gain plan exactly. Expect to fluctuate. Some weeks you may only gain half a pound and then the next week gain two.

> "But the goal of every pregnant woman should be to keep weight gain as steady as possible, without any sudden jumps or drops." (Eisenberg, Murkoff, and Hathaway, *What to Expect When You're Expecting*, Workman, 1996, p. 148)

When Should You Be Concerned about Your Weight During Pregnancy?

Regular weigh-ins at your doctor's should keep you on track. However, you should be concerned if you think you have been eating sensibly and any of the following occurs:

- You gain more than seven pounds a month
- You gain less than half a pound a month after the first trimester
- You don't gain any weight for two weeks or more during the fourth to eighth months
- You gain more than three pounds in any one week in the second trimester
- You gain more than two pounds a week in the third trimester
- You gain no weight for two weeks in a row

Any of the above could indicate that fetal development is not progressing at a normal rate and the health of your baby-to-be as well as yourself is at risk. Your doctor should be able to determine the cause—but if your weight does go astray because of overeating or an inadequate intake of calories, you need to talk to your doctor to discuss how you can get back on track. He or she will evaluate where you are now and the weight you still need to gain for your baby.

Remember that for every day in your pregnancy, your baby needs a steady supply of nutrients. Never, ever, *ever* put your baby-to-be on a diet to stop you getting fat.

Disordered Eating
and Pregnancy

FOR MANY WOMEN, WEIGHT GAIN DURING PREGNANCY PRESENTS A challenge to self-image. Body image is closely linked to a sense of self. How we look expresses who we are, and the bodily changes and weight gain of pregnancy can be difficult to come to terms with. But most of us manage to deal with it. After all, we are pregnant. Women who suffer from eating disorders, however, can't shrug the weight gain off. For them the only important thing in life is to be thin. There is a terror of gaining weight. Fat is seen as repulsive. Ritualistic behavior controls how they eat. They weigh themselves repeatedly. For women who suffer or have suffered from eating disorders, such as anorexia or bulimia or abuse of laxatives and diuretics to lose weight, the natural weight gain of pregnancy can be a terrifying ordeal.

"Before I got pregnant I weighed 105 pounds. This was still not quite the weight I wanted to be. I wanted to be 100 pounds. I'm 5 feet 5 inches. At four months I started to lose my waistline. I was terrified. I just stopped eating. I didn't think I was harming the baby. I thought she would get what she needed." Rebecca, age 19

"My doctor hospitalized me in the sixth month when I failed to put on enough weight. I had only gained ten pounds and was underweight before I got pregnant." Sarah, age 20

"I suffered from an eating disorder. Being pregnant is incredibly hard for me. I feel repulsive when I gain weight." Demi, age 31

"I want a baby, but don't think I could face gaining all that weight." Belinda, age 36

A woman with anorexia tries to starve herself into a dangerously malnourished condition that she often manages to hide with loose and baggy clothes. Even when very thin, she sees herself as overweight and is terrified of gaining any weight. She is willing to sacrifice anything to stay thin, and that may include a fetus should she get pregnant.

In a similar way to the anorexic, a bulimic is obsessed with body image. With bulimia, though, a woman binges on a massive amount of food and then vomits or uses laxatives or diuretics to bring it back up. She may also go on very strict diets and exercise excessively. Bulimia is a secretive disorder. Often a bulimic woman may appear normal in weight, but maintains her weight with bizarre eating patterns.

Obesity is another dangerous eating disorder, although at the opposite end of the control spectrum. It can put the health of mom and baby-to-be at risk, but only when weight is truly excessive for height and build.

Nearly 80 percent of women who get eating disorders are young and in their reproductive years. What happens when they get pregnant? According to an insightful article by Pamela Warrick called "Time to Heal" in *Fit Pregnancy* (Winter 1997, p. 98) "Atlanta certified eating-disorders specialist Julie Dryden DeLettre, M.H.S., has seen a growing trend of women with eating disorders becoming pregnant. She and other professionals in the field believe that doctors are not recognizing the underlying anorexia or bulimia that causes these women to be so underweight."

In most cases women with eating disorders have difficulties becoming pregnant because eating disorders can disturb the normal functioning of hormones. However, in some cases pregnancy does occur. Pregnancy can also become a particularly vulnerable time for women who have had eating disorders in the past and who have managed to get their diet under control. Pregnancy causes old fears to resurface and old behavior patterns to reestablish themselves. According to Shaila Misri, M.D., author of *Shouldn't I Be Happy?*

(Free Press, 1995, p. 19), "The majority of eating disorders in pregnancy represents the continuation of pre-existing disorders. Very few cases of a woman experiencing an eating disorder for the first time during pregnancy have been reported."

So far there has been no definitive statement on the cause of eating disorders, and most experts agree that many factors contribute to the development of the disorder. Some explain it physically: a genetic disease, a defect in the brain, an imbalance in body chemistry, a metabolic problem, a problem with how the nervous system processes messages about appetite, a hormonal imbalance, and so on. Others believe that the powerful popular stereotypes of the ideal feminine image contribute to the development of eating disorders. Being extremely thin is not how nature intended us to be.

Others see it more as a psychological problem caused by self-hatred or conflict within families or with loved ones. By remaining in an adolescent body type, a woman can avoid conflicts about her sexual identity or the demands of sexual maturity. Erratic and unhealthy eating habits are often a way of coping with difficult emotional passages. And pregnancy is one of the most challenging emotional passages a woman can face. Perhaps the struggle with food expresses ambivalent feelings about becoming pregnant. Is the baby really wanted? Is there a secure relationship? Is pregnancy being used as an excuse to avoid facing other issues in your life? Is there a fear of motherhood, of responsibility? Is the understanding of what being a woman means so damaged that baby-to-be's health is put at risk?

Whatever the cause, severe cases of anorexia, bulimia, or obesity during pregnancy often require hospitalization, counseling, and medication. Alongside medication, psychological counseling will be needed on a long-term basis so that inappropriate behavior can be recognized and a new self-image adjusted to. A dietitian should play an important role in treatment, as should a supportive counselor. Treatment of eating disorders during pregnancy, whether full-blown or borderline, must include physical therapy as well as counseling. The emotional and the physical need to addressed if recovery is to be complete.

A woman who allows an eating disorder to continue during pregnancy can create serious health problems for herself and her unborn baby. It is vital that she get help. "Even with the most positive attitude toward the pregnancy and expected child, women with eating disorders are seldom able to alter their self-destructive behavior on their own. They need both the sympathetic awareness of and support from their families, and also the professional resources of trained counselors to assist them." (Dr. Shaila Misri, *Shouldn't I Be Happy?*, Free Press, 1995, p. 20)

If an eating disorder persists, baby-to-be is not getting the best diet for development. Mom is lacking the nutrients she needs to nourish herself and baby-to-be. Premature birth is the greatest risk if a woman is very underweight. Baby is also likely to be a very low birth weight. The smaller and more premature a baby is, the harder it is for it to survive. In the words of Dr. Jacobs, "You always want a baby to gain enough to have the best chances of survival."

The Renfrew Center is a women's mental health facility in Coconut Creek, Florida. It specializes in eating disorders, and it has come up with some alarming statistics about how an eating disorder can affect a baby. Anorexics and bulimics have an average weight gain of between six and sixteen pounds during pregnancy. Babies born tend to be around five pounds. For women with eating disorders, prenatal mortality is nearly six times greater and incidence of low birth weight babies around two times greater than expected rates.

Pregnancy Can Heal

Although there has been relatively little published research on the subject, several recent studies of small groups of pregnant women with eating disorders suggest that pregnancy seems to heal if only temporarily what ails anorexic and bulimic women. (*Fit Pregnancy*, Winter 1997, p. 101)

Why this happens is not clear. Perhaps the hormonal changes of pregnancy can have a beneficial effect and give a woman with eating disorder a new sense of purpose. Barbara Friedman, M.E.D., conducted a survey on pregnancy and eating disorders. Her survey, which seems to be backed up by other research, shows that pregnancy can improve body image for women with eating disorders. It is socially acceptable to be gaining weight when you are pregnant. Friedman also noticed that pregnancy was a time when women acknowledged for the first time that they had a problem and needed help, now that someone else's life was at stake and not just their own. Eating disorders are often associated with feelings of loneliness, depression, and a sense of emptiness. For some women, having a baby can fill that void. For a while at least, attention shifts from oneself to baby. "And let's not discount the simple natural desire to be a good mother, a good caretaker," says Jean Rubel, Ph.D., who founded an information clearing house on eating disorders, ANRED (Anorexia Nervosa and Related Eating Disorders). "I have heard eating disordered mothers say something as straightforward as 'I want to be warmer and softer for my baby. I don't want him to feel like he's hugging a bicycle.'" (Quoted from *Fit Pregnancy*, Winter 1997, p. 118)

For many women with eating disorders, pregnancy is a time to heal and construct a more healthy body image and attitude toward food. According to Hartley Gise, M.D., clinical professor of psychiatry for the John A. Burns School of Medicine at the University of Hawaii, "Pregnancy can help many women with eating disorders recover." But he also points out that "it is important to remember that eating disorders are 'an illness that can be successfully treated; it's not just a weakness you can talk yourself out of.'" (Quoted from "Time to Heal," Pamela Warrick, *Fit Pregnancy*, Winter 1997, p. 118.) Research indicates that even though pregnancy can bring healing, the healing tends to be temporary. Once baby is born, symptoms often return. Disordered eating can become a way of dealing with the demands of life with a baby—the stress and chaos of being a mom.

If you have severe eating problems, the first step on the road to recovery is recognizing that you are suffering from an illness and not just some kind of personality defect or weakness. You need help. If you have a history of problems with food and body image, talk to your doctor. Your doctor can then advise or refer you to someone else or to help in your community. There is help out there—even safe medications that can be taken when you are pregnant to make sure you and your baby-to-be stay well. "Your own mental health is important to you and your baby. Make it your first priority." (Quoted from *Fit Pregnancy*, Winter 1997, p. 118.)

Seek advice from your doctor if you have a history of eating disorders and you are pregnant.

Borderline Eating Disorders

"I don't think about what is healthy, so much as what can I eat that is low in calories. I am very strict with my calories. I never go over 1,800 a day. I'm five months pregnant." Julia, age 27

"I skipped lunch today because I couldn't jog for my usual forty-five minutes this morning. I'm three months pregnant." Stephanie, age 29

Full-blown eating disorders such as anorexia and bulimia tend to receive the most attention because of their shock value. For years now we have got used to hearing about them. Lost in the shuffle, however, are women with less severe cases of dysfunctional eating. "They don't take it so far, but they hate their bodies just as much," says Joanne Stuart, M.S., R.D., of Health Training Resources, a nutritional counseling firm in Branford, Connecticut (*Shape*, March 1998, p. 99).

Obsessive eating is defined by Frances Berg, editor of *Healthy Weight Journal*, in terms of how much time you spend thinking about food and weight. In *Afraid to Eat: Children and Teens in Weight Crisis* (Healthy Weight Publishing Network, 1997), Berg says women with eating disorders think about food 90 percent of the time. Dysfunctional eaters think about food 20 to 60 percent of the time. A poor body image is often combined with dysfunctional eating and exercising obsessively. These women exercise to burn calories, not to feel healthy. Their diets are dysfunctional in an effort to keep weight low, but not dangerously low. There is an irrational fear of gaining weight. "They base their happiness and sadly their sense of self worth on their food and exercise choices." (*Shape*, March 1998, p. 99)

Do you recognize yourself here? If you do, then you fall into a category that health professionals have trouble identifying, the shadowy world of borderline eating disorders. The condition is probably very common. You may not even know you have it. Millions and millions of us obsess about our weight. We diet strictly. We exercise. We count calories. We get upset if we put on a few pounds. We wish we could lose weight. We feel more confident about ourselves if we lose weight.

Dysfunctional eating is dangerous. It could even develop into a full-blown eating disorder. If you have poor eating habits and you exercise obsessively to lose weight, the costs to your health are high: nutritional deficiencies, injuries, and often depression are likely. You probably won't lose much weight, either, as your body rebels with a slow metabolism. If you are pregnant, the cost to your health and that of your baby-to-be is even higher. Neither of you will be getting the nutrients you both need.

The important thing is to get help if you are having real problems with food and eating. Part Two will give recommendations about weight management during pregnancy but you may need extra help. The resources section at the end of this book offers some useful addresses to contact. But if your diet is spiraling out of control, if you can't cope with the weight gain of pregnancy, see a doctor or talk to a counselor or nutritionist. Ask for help and ask for it now.

No woman should be pregnant and hating it.

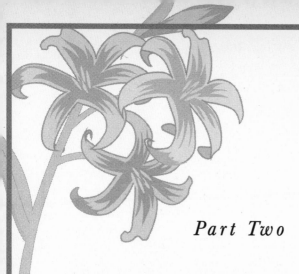

Part Two

Weight Management During Pregnancy

*"Since I've been pregnant, my breasts,
my rear end, and even my feet have grown.
Is there anything that gets smaller during pregnancy?"
"Yes—your bladder."*

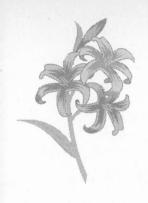

6

Eating Like a Grown-Up

WHETHER YOU ARE READY OR NOT, IN LESS THAN NINE MONTHS YOU WILL become a parent. That means eating like a grown-up.

Many women have very erratic eating habits. We eat on the go. We skip breakfast. We have a cappuccino for lunch. We have a Snickers bar to keep our energy going. We go out in the evening to a fine meal with wine. We diet. We indulge. We try to stick to a healthy eating plan. We succumb to a chocolate binge. Somehow we get by.

> "I had chips for lunch. Is the carbohydrate good for me? I know I shouldn't have had them. I do feel guilty."

> "I'm going to breastfeed and I'll lose all the weight I gain. I'm eating for two and that means I can eat what I want when I want."

> "It's going to be strange to have to sit down to three well-balanced meals a day."

> "How am I going to be able to make sure I am eating right?"

> "Well, as long as I take the diet supplements my doctor gave me I should be OK."

> "Chocolate isn't that bad for you. Ice cream has calcium in it."

> "French fries, double cheeseburger, and diet Pepsi, please. I'm eating for two."

When I got pregnant I was forced to look at what I was actually eating.

A typical day might have been something like this:

No breakfast. Latte. No lunch. Midafternoon snack like a cake, scone, cereal, or chocolate bar, and another latte. In the evening I'd eat a huge salad with bread and cheese. Before I went to bed, a bowl of cereal. During the day I'd suck sweets, chew gum, and drink diet Pepsi.

Once I was pregnant, I knew I just couldn't live like that anymore. The food you eat provides the material for your tissues and organs. You are what you eat. And when you get pregnant, baby-to-be is what you eat, too. "You cannot hope to grow a baby if you do not have the building blocks stored in your body or do not supply them in your dietary intake." (Gillespie, *Your Pregnancy*, Harper Perennial, 1992, p. 66)

Basically, I was going to have to learn about food and nutrition. I was going to have to learn to eat properly. I had to set a good example for my child. I reached for as many pregnancy diet books as I could find. Suddenly food became an important issue. I wanted to eat right. I wanted to get all my nutrients. I wanted to eat enough to gain the right amount of weight for me.

It was not easy. Everybody seemed interested in what I was eating now. I felt intense pressure not only from myself, but from friends and family. As I sat down to a meal, "Is that good for the baby?" was written across everybody's face as I filled my plate. There were keen observations on every morsel I ate. Discerning eyes never failed to torture me when I ate too much pizza or ice cream.

And I got so much conflicting advice: Eat a lot. Eat a little. Take supplements. Don't take supplements. Eat what you want. Don't eat what you want. Drink four glasses of milk a day. Avoid milk. You can eat chocolate. Don't eat chocolate. Drink six to eight glasses a day of water, and on and on and on.

It was overwhelming. Eating was hard work. Trying to drink those six to eight glasses of water made me feel dizzy. I hated the food I was eating. I felt miserable. I felt like I was doing everything wrong. I was never going to eat right. In a fit of despair I went and had a chocolate scone and then another one. I was tempted to just rely on the diet supplements my doctor had given me. But they made me feel sick. I could taste them all morning. Worse still, they made me constipated.

Things were going to have to change. I didn't want to be anxious about food for the rest of my pregnancy. I wanted to give my baby what he needed. I also didn't want to gain more weight than I needed. It was up to me to find a way to eat for two that worked for both of us.

Ask Your Body What It Needs

Something I read in the *Pregnant Woman's Comfort Book* really struck a chord.

> A doctor said to a pregnant friend, "I wish all women could think about food like a pregnant woman." What the doctor meant was a pregnant body speaks up very loudly telling you what it needs. (Jennifer Louden, Harper San Francisco, 1995, p. 105)

Louden is right. If you can be patient with yourself and ask your body what it needs, you will be amazed. You will just know what your body and your baby-to-be needs to eat. When you are pregnant you become very attuned to your body's needs. You know when you are hungry. You know what kinds of foods will make you sick. You know what you can manage to eat and what you can't.

But I also knew that sometimes I got confused and didn't know how to listen to my bodily wisdom. My mood, how rushed I was, what time of day it was, what food store I was shopping in, influenced my food choices. On many occasions I didn't know how to follow my intuition. There were times when I thought my body really needed chocolate and needed it now. But was that right for my baby-to-be? Probably not.

Despite wanting to follow my bodily wisdom, I definitely needed some solid nutritional advice to help me make the right decisions. For so long now I had been turning to food for comfort when I was tired, stressed, or emotional. Now that I was pregnant, I had to learn to balance the risk to my baby-to-be against my need. I talked to my doctor and got some advice on nutrition during pregnancy. She suggested I keep a food diary so that I could check what I was eating. She stressed how important taking a diet supplement was to ensure I got all the vitamins and minerals I needed in case my diet fell short.

Looking back, I can see that when I started to make the right choices for my baby-to-be, I was also making the right choices for me. It was during my pregnancy that I really started to make healthy, grown-up decisions about the food I was eating. It felt good.

And in weighing the baby's need against my own and finding a compromise between the two that was right for both of us, I was also getting my first lesson in parenthood.

A Healthy Diet

The single most important factor in excessive weight gain during pregnancy is poor diet. Women's dietary habits are getting worse and worse. Fewer and fewer of us stick to a healthy diet. The incidence of eating disorders is high. Research on the nutritional status of pregnant women and mothers suggests that their diets lack nutrients, vitamins, and minerals. The infant survival rate in America is poor compared to many other countries. (Denmark has the highest infant survival rate.) One of the major reasons for this is poor diet. The American diet is perhaps one of the most unhealthy in the world: high in fat and sugar and fast food with little nutritional value. Obesity is already a problem in this country.

The quality of the food you eat is far more important than the quantity. Too much junk food will result in an excessive weight gain whether you are pregnant or not. If your goal during pregnancy is to gain nutritiously, have a healthy baby, and also manage your weight so you don't put on more than is needed, a healthy diet is essential. A healthy diet includes all the essential nutrients our bodies need: protein, carbohydrates, fat, vitamins, minerals, and water. The demands for certain nutrients increases during pregnancy (see Figure 6), and these will be outlined below.

Eating right during pregnancy is much easier than you might think. All that is needed is a bit of dietary common sense. "There's no mystical, magical miracle diet for pregnancy; it's fairly simple." (Connie Marshall, *From Here to Maternity*, Conmar, 1997, p. 21)

The following diet recommendations have been adapted from the U.S. Department of Agriculture Guide to Daily Food Choices and the Recommended Daily Allowances (RDAs) of the Food and Nutrition Board of the National Academy of Sciences.

FIGURE 6: ESSENTIAL NUTRIENTS DURING PREGNANCY

NUTRIENT	RDA	SOURCES	WHY NEEDED
Vitamin A	800 mcg RE	Dark green vegetables, eggs	Immune system, vision, cell and tissue growth
Vitamin C	70 mg	Green leafy vegetables, peas	Cell function, connective tissue, bones, teeth, blood vessels
Vitamin D	10 mcg	Cereal, fortified milk, salmon	Strong bones in baby and mom
Vitamin E	10 mg	Wheat germ, nuts, spinach	Protection from damage caused by free radicals
Vitamin K	65 mcg	Broccoli, tomatoes, bananas	Blood clotting and bone formation
Vitamin B6	2.2 mg	Fish, potatoes, bananas	Baby's brain and nerve tissue
Vitamin B12	2.2 mcg	Fish, eggs, milk, meat	Cell growth
Thiamine (B1)	1.5 mg	Peanuts, green leafy vegetables	Nervous system, growth of body and brain
Riboflavin (B2)	1.6 mg	Milk, green leafy vegetables	All tissue growth
Niacin (B3)	17 mg	Chicken, fish, peanut butter	Tissue growth, nerves, digestion
Folic a cid	400 mcg	Green leafy vegetables, broccoli, peas	Cell division, prevents birth defects, normal growth
Calcium	1,200 mg	Milk, tofu, green leafy vegetables	Formation of baby's bones and maintenance of mom's
Iodine	175 mcg	Seafood, vegetables	Normal growth and development
Iron	30 mg	Red meat, peas, broccoli	Transport of oxygen, enzyme function
Magnesium	320 mg	Peanuts, spinach, potatoes	Strong bones and healthy nerves
Phosphorus	1,200 mg	Grains, nuts, legumes, milk	Metabolism
Selenium	65 mcg	Cereals, seafood, eggs	Removal of harmful products
Zinc	15 mg	Animal products, seeds, nuts	Cell function and development
Protein	60 g	Meat, fish, eggs, milk, cheese	Formation of baby's tissue, placenta, and red blood cells in mom

RDA = Recommended Daily Allowance
RE = Retinol equivalents
mg = milligrams
mcg = micrograms

Nutritional needs increase during pregnancy—compare with Figure 12 (RDA for nonpregnant woman)

Warning—Vitamin A and vitamin E are toxic in large amounts.

PROTEIN

Proteins are the substances that build tissues for growth and repair for you and your baby-to-be. Proteins are especially important when you are pregnant and during lactation when new tissues are forming. The typical American diet tends to be very high in protein. Although protein is vital for healthy growth and development, too much can make you feel listless. It is not a good source of energy. When you are pregnant you need about 70–100 grams of protein a day. You should aim to make it about 25 percent of your diet. Good food sources of protein include vegetables, legumes, and other plant sources. Other sources include lean meat, skinned chicken and fish, eggs, milk, cheese, peanuts, and skim milk.

If you are a vegetarian, you can still get enough protein and have a healthy baby. But you need to be even more careful when you plan your diet and ensure that you get enough protein. Eggs and milk products should be sufficient. If you are a vegan, you need vegetable proteins and meat substitutes. (Vegans must make sure they get adequate calcium. Vegetarians should ensure that they get enough vitamin B12 and folic acid and vitamin D. If you find this hard to do in your diet, it is essential that you take a dietary supplement when you are pregnant.)

CARBOHYDRATES

Carbohydrates are your main source of energy. They are divided into two groups: starches and sugars. Starches (complex carbohydrates) are a steady source of energy and will satisfy your hunger. Sugars won't, and they should be eaten sparingly. Good complex carbohydrates are whole-grain bread, pasta, vegetables, grains, and fruit. They are not too fattening, but watch out for the fattening dressings you may put on them.

Carbohydrates, like fruit, contain fiber, which is important for keeping your digestive system running smoothly. Carbohydrates should be about half of your daily diet. Remember, though—if you consume too much, they will be not be used as energy but stored as fat. This is even more true for sugars such as chocolate, cakes, and candy.

FAT

Fats keep your body functioning and are an important energy source. They are also an important source of vitamins A and D. Don't cut fat out of your diet when you get pregnant. A diet too low in fat is not healthy. You need to make fat about 25 percent of your diet. Eating too much fat, though, is not good either. Weight will pile on as fat is only used for energy when you run short of carbohydrates.

Avoid saturated fat, which is usually of animal origin, if you can. It is too high in cholesterol. Look for polyunsaturated fats. The best thing to do is to read the labels of the fats you buy. Corn and vegetable oil should be used in cooking as well as in sauces and dressings.

Vitamins and Minerals

If your diet does not have the vitamins and minerals you need, your body won't be able to properly absorb the nutrients it needs. For example, if you lack sufficient Vitamin B, your body won't be able to use the fats, proteins, and carbohydrates properly. Vitamin C helps your body absorb iron. Zinc aids digestion. So if you don't give your body the vitamins and minerals it needs, not only do you put your baby-to-be's health at risk, but problems with weight management are likely to occur.

Let's briefly look at the most important vitamins and minerals your body needs, and then see how these needs increase when you are pregnant.

VITAMINS

Vitamin A fights infection and prevents dry skin and poor bone growth. It is found in vegetables, milk, butter, margarine, and egg yolk.

Vitamin B1 (thiamine) is important for carbon dioxide removal during respiration. It is found in whole-grain, nuts, and seeds.

Vitamin B2 (riboflavin) is needed for growth and is in milk, meat, eggs, and leafy vegetables.

Vitamin B3 (niacin) is an aid in preventing disease, improving mood, and for a glowing complexion. You can find it in milk, eggs, cheeses, and fish.

Vitamin B5 (pantothenic acid) is essential for energy metabolism and is found in many foods.

Vitamin B6 is important for the metabolism of proteins. It is found in spinach, broccoli, and bananas.

Vitamin B12 for healthy skin and nervous system is in meat, milk, eggs, cheese, and fish.

Biotin is important for carbohydrate and fat metabolism. It is found in liver, peanuts, and cheese.

Folic acid (folate) is for cell production and healthy skin and is in leafy green vegetables, chicken, liver, and kidney.

Vitamin C, found in green vegetables and citrus fruits, prevents colds, heals wounds, and is essential for normal metabolism. It boosts the immune system and protects us from toxins.

Vitamin D is for bone growth and calcium absorption. It is found in tuna fish, eggs, butter, and cheese. It is also produced by our skins when we are exposed to sunlight.

Vitamin E promotes blood clotting and is found in milk, vegetables, liver, rice, and bran.

Vitamin K is active in maintaining the involuntary nervous system, vascular system, and involuntary muscles. It is in wheat germ, vegetable oil, and whole-grain breads and cereals.

MINERALS

Calcium is for bone growth, healthy teeth, blood clotting, and iron absorption and is an aid for relieving menstrual problems. It is found in milk, milk products, egg yolk, green vegetables, and shellfish.

Copper is an aid for the metabolism of iron and is found in liver and whole grains.

Fluoride strengthens teeth and is found in fluoridated water and tea.

Iron is the basic component of blood hemoglobin and prevents anemia. It is found in meat, green vegetables, yeast, and wheat germ.

Iodine is found in seafood and seaweed and is an aid in regulating energy use in the body.

Magnesium, found in milk, grains, vegetables, fruits, and cereals, is involved in the normal functioning of the brain, spinal cord, and nerves and is an aid in bone formation.

Potassium is needed for healthy nerves and muscles and is found in milk, fruit, and vegetables.

Sodium maintains adequate water in cells in the body and is found in table salt, milk, and meat.

Phosphorus, found in milk, yogurt, yeast, and wheat germ, is required for bone growth, strong teeth, and energy transformation.

Zinc plays an essential role in the development of reproductive organs and in the body's enzyme systems. It is found in egg yolk, milk, nuts, peas, and beans.

When you are pregnant, getting your vitamins and minerals has never been so important. They are essential for the normal development and growth of your baby-to-be as well as for you. The body can't store or produce its own vitamins and minerals. You must get them from the food you eat. A normal balanced diet should give you what you need, but if you have a poor diet, it is very easy to become deficient in them as a result. Consult your doctor about the use of any supplements or over-the-counter medications. (See the section in the next chapter on dietary supplements.)

During pregnancy the requirements for certain vitamins and minerals increases:

- Your folic acid requirement doubles when you are pregnant. High intake before conception may help reduce the chances of neural defects in your baby. Women who take a 400-microgram supplement of folic acid prior to conception and for the first eight weeks are thought to avoid fetal abnormalities. Higher doses than this, though, should not be taken.
- Vitamin A is dangerous in large amounts. Amounts over 800 micrograms RE can be toxic. Take natural beta carotene (4,000 IU daily) instead.
- Vitamin C is needed for tissue repair, metabolism, and wound healing. Your baby needs it for healthy teeth and bones. Your body can't produce vitamin C, so you need a constant daily supply. Vitamin C aids iron absorption. Seventy milligrams daily is recommended. Good sources are fruit, tomatoes, red and green peppers, broccoli, cauliflower, spinach, and strawberries.
- Vitamin D. You need 10 micrograms daily for calcium absorption and bone formation. Your requirement for vitamin D doubles when you are pregnant. It can be toxic in large doses, though.
- Vitamin E. You need 10 milligrams daily. Premature and low birth weight infants are often deficient in vitamin E. Excessive amounts are harmful.

- Iron is important because it helps red blood cells carry oxygen in the blood. You could get anemia if you have too little, so make sure you are not deficient. Iron also helps the functions of many enzymes in the body. You and your baby need it. Good food sources of iron include liver, breads and cereals, dried peas and beans, broccoli, and spinach. Get 30 milligrams daily or as directed by your doctor. Take with 100 milligrams of vitamin C for better absorption.

- Calcium is crucial for the development and maintenance of your skeleton, and for nerve cell and muscle function, for blood clotting, and many other cellular functions. Your calcium needs rise during pregnancy, especially in the last trimester. If you are lacking vitamin D, this will affect the amount of calcium you have in your blood. Your growing baby needs calcium to build strong bones and teeth. If you are calcium deficient, your baby will drain calcium from your bones and you could suffer from osteoporosis later in life. You need about 1,200–1,300 milligrams a day. Good food sources include dairy products and leafy vegetables. Almonds, peanuts, and dried fruit are also good sources. A good source of calcium is milk and milk products. If you can drink milk, you will get all the calcium you need from four eight-ounce glasses a day. If you hate milk or have lactose tolerance problems, yogurt, lactose-free products, and green leafy vegetables are alternatives. Milk should be skim or fat-free.

- Magnesium: You need 320 milligrams daily to balance with calcium.

- Iodine is needed for the thyroid hormones that help your baby grow and develop normally. If you are deficient, it could impair your baby's physical and emotional development. Good food sources are seafood and vegetables.

- Zinc is important for healthy cell function and for your baby's development. During pregnancy, zinc requirements increase. Insufficient zinc intake is linked to low birth weight. Good food sources include nuts, whole-grain cereal, legumes, liver, and eggs. You should aim for 15 milligrams daily. Don't go over 75 milligrams.

- Selenium helps remove harmful products produced in your body. Good food sources include seafood, eggs, and cereal.

Water

And finally, don't forget the most important nutrient that your body needs—water. Our bodies are about two-thirds water, so the intake and distribution of fluid is vital. If the body is deprived of water, blood volume is reduced and does not circulate to your tissues and to the fetus as effectively. You will feel dizzy and fatigued if you are dehydrated. Your needs increase when you are pregnant because of metabolic requirements and loss of fluids.

The solution is to drink enough water. Six to eight glasses a day is the recommended amount when you are pregnant. If that seems like hard work, try juices. Adding a slice of lemon to water also helps. Soft drinks are fine, but make sure they are free of sugar and caffeine. Remember, though, that soft drinks contain sodium, which may give you fluid retention.

To see if you are drinking enough water, check the color of your urine. If it is too dark, you are dehydrated. It should be a light yellow, the color of water with one lemon added.

Nutritional Hints

Find out how much you are actually eating. Keep a food diary, and start to become aware of the foods you eat. See how nutritious your food choices are.

If you are not eating enough fruit and vegetables and whole grains, make sure you include them in your diet. An excellent source of vitamins and minerals for your body is green leafy vegetables and fresh fruit. If you add dressings, keep to oil dressings and vinegar-based dressings. Try to eat green vegetables and yellow fruits every day as well as other fruits and vegetables. Legumes and whole grain, such as whole-grain bread, brown rice, and whole-grain cereal, are also beneficial. Cereal can be a healthy food choice, but look for cereals that are high in carbohydrate and fiber, like shredded wheat, and not those like granola that are high in fat and sugar.

As far as sugar and salt are concerned, eat them in moderation. Salt won't give you toxemia or hypertension unless you eat far too much. It might give you bloating, though. You can have a few teaspoons of sugar a day and it won't harm you or your baby. The odd chocolate bar and scoop of ice cream will not ruin your diet. Moderation is the key. Foods like chocolate and cookies are very high in sugar. Eating too many of them will add on the pounds. Watch out for hidden sugars in many of the other foods you eat, too. Read labels. If you want to use sweeteners, no conclusive studies have shown that they are harmful.

Foods to avoid during pregnancy include "junk food," highly seasoned food, coffee, fried foods, and rare or undercooked meat, poultry, or fish. Especially avoid raw eggs, raw meat, and unpasteurized foods like soft cheese. (Some cheese contain harmful bacteria. Avoid mold-ripened cheeses, such as brie and all blue cheeses; unpasteurized sheep's and goat's cheese should also be given a miss. Cottage cheese and hard cheeses, however, are fine and a good source of protein and calcium.) Grilling can produce harmful substances in meat so avoid grilled meats. Reducing or eliminating the amount of caffeine and alcohol is essential. Alcohol is harmful to your unborn child and can cause high blood pressure; caffeine can cause stress, fatigue, headaches, and lack of energy for the mom-to-be. Caffeine and alcohol also deplete the body of water and minerals because they have a diuretic effect. Cigarettes and drugs are also damaging. You and your baby-to-be don't need them.

Now that you've read all about a healthy diet, don't get despondent if yours doesn't match up. Few, if any, pregnant women eat a perfect diet when they are pregnant. Despite this, they have perfectly healthy pregnancies and babies. I have yet to meet the woman who for every day of her pregnancy establishes the correct percentage of carbohydrate, protein, and fat, drinks all that water, eats all those vegetables and fruit, and gets exactly the right amount of vitamins and minerals. The great majority of us just do the best that we can. We get through the nine months somehow!

Don't become obsessive about your diet, but use this information as a sort of guideline for you to refer to or to get you back on track. Knowledge about what a healthy diet actually is and what nutrients you need will make you more aware of what you are eating. Armed with this knowledge, you can make food choices that make sense for you and baby-to-be. Dietary common sense is all that is needed for most of us to eat a healthy diet. Dietary common sense is also an integral part of weight management during and after pregnancy.

Now we have looked at what we should be eating when we are pregnant, let's now take a look at how much we should be eating. Should we be "eating for two"?

7

Eating for Two?

WHEN YOU GET PREGNANT, YOU HAVE TO EAT FOR TWO. IF YOU HAVE struggled with dieting for years, this might seem like a ticket to paradise.

And now for the bad news: Although true in some respects, the "eating for two" tradition is what causes many weight management problems during pregnancy and postpartum. Eating for two does not mean what most of us think it means, i.e., eating twice as much as usual. Let's explain.

A calorie is a unit of energy that is given off by a certain amount of food when it is burned or used by your body. I'm sure I don't need to tell you that different types of foods have different calorie values. The ones we like usually tend to be high in calories! Lettuce has virtually no calories, but a chocolate bar has hundreds. You could eat as much lettuce as you like and not gain a pound. Eat all the chocolate you like and you will wear it on your hips.

Depending on your build and how active you are, the number of calories required for the average medium-framed nonpregnant woman who is moderately active is in the range of 2,000 to 2,400 daily. Calorie requirements when you are pregnant will increase because you need energy for two—yourself and the baby-to-be. But they won't increase that much.

It takes about 55,000 calories to make a baby. That might seem a lot, but it is equivalent to around 300 extra calories a day (a glass of low-fat milk, an apple, and a slice of bread, for example), and that's only in the last two trimesters.

Time and time again women realize too late that they have misunderstood what eating for two means. "They think they can eat as much as they like because they are feeding two. But they end up eating a lot more than is actually necessary. What your body and your baby-to-be doesn't need is stored as fat." (Dr. Jacobs) Weight management problems after pregnancy are usually related to gaining more weight than you needed when you were pregnant. If you can manage to stay within the range recommended for your height and build, you could save yourself a lot of grief postpartum. Having five or ten pounds to lose is far easier than having twenty or thirty pounds to lose.

If you are pregnant and you know you have gained too much, don't try to lose weight now. Your baby-to-be must have a constant supply of fresh nutrients from you every day. Talk to your doctor and make sure that your calorie intake is not in excess of what you and your baby-to-be need. For the average woman, that means about 2,300 to 2,700 calories a day. Adjust your diet accordingly.

How Much Should You Eat Each Day?

Food guides can not only help you assess the nutritional quality of your diet, but they can also help you find out if you are eating too much or too little. Remember, though—they are not perfect. As scientists discover new information, food guides change and nutritionists revise their opinions. At present the bread, rice, cereal, and pasta food group recommendation is six to eleven servings a day; the fruit group, two to four servings a day; the vegetable group three to five servings a day; and the milk, yogurt, and cheese group, two to three servings daily. For meat, poultry, fish, eggs, and nuts, two to three servings a day are recommended, with fats, oils, and sweets to be eaten sparingly. (See Figure 7.)

FIGURE 7: USDA FOOD GUIDE TO DAILY SERVINGS

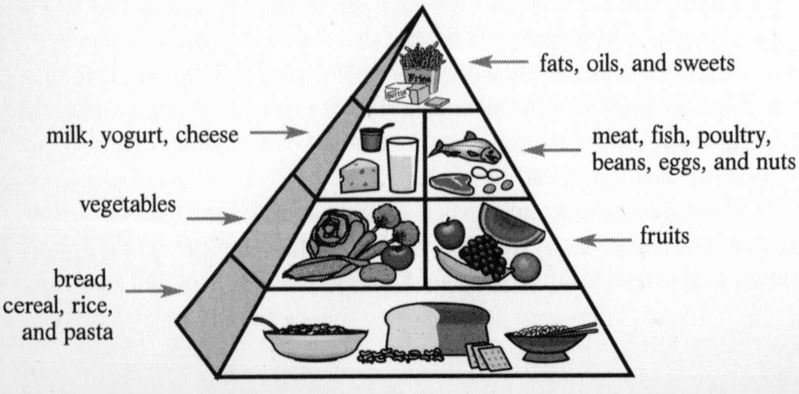

fats, oils, and sweets

milk, yogurt, cheese

meat, fish, poultry, beans, eggs, and nuts

vegetables

fruits

bread, cereal, rice, and pasta

When you are pregnant, the daily food guide to ensure optimum nutrition and calorie intake a day during pregnancy would look something like this:

Have at least six servings of whole grains such as whole-wheat bread and crackers, whole-grain cereal, brown rice, potatoes, and oatmeal. (One serving is one slice of bread.) This gives you fiber to keep you regular; carbohydrates to fuel the metabolic processes and cell divisions that make your baby; B vitamins that contribute to growth and give you energy; magnesium for building bones and nerves; other trace minerals like copper that are important in preventing birth defects and aid in the development of connective tissue vital for baby's skeletal, nervous and circulatory systems; and finally, folic acid, a B vitamin that will prevent neural tube defects and preterm delivery.

Have lots of fresh fruit and vegetables—around nine or ten servings a day of fresh, plain frozen, or canned vegetables, or fruits that are fresh or canned in their own juice, such as orange, grapefruit, or tomato juice. This gives you not only folic acid, but also antioxidant nutrients such as vitamin C and beta carotene that protect you and your baby from the damage caused by free radicals. They also help with cell division and the formation of connective tissue, including skin.

If you can, have at least four servings of milk and milk products. (One serving is one cup of milk or yogurt, one ounce of cheese, or two cups of cottage cheese.) These foods include low-fat or nonfat milk, low-fat yogurt, hard cheese, cottage cheese, and soy milk with vitamins and calcium. This gives you calcium, which prevents lead mobilization from bone tissue and, along with Vitamin D, builds strong bones; vitamin B12 and B6 to aid in nerve development; and protein for the formation of enzymes, nerve chemicals, and muscle tissue.

A large percentage of the population, however, have sensitivities to milk and milk products that run beyond lactose intolerance, including upper respiratory tract congestion, mood changes, and general lack of ability to digest, which puts a strain on the whole body. Anyone who has to safeguard their energy is usually advised by Chinese doctors to limit dairy products. Milk is a readily available source of calcium, so it is often recommended, but there are other ways of getting enough calcium. You might be able to tolerate certain kinds of dairy foods, such as hard cheese or lactose-reduced milk, but if you need to avoid dairy products altogether, you can still get all the calcium your baby-to-be needs from other nondairy foods such as soy milk and soy protein, broccoli, dried fruit, dried beans, almonds, and baked goods made with sesame seeds, soy flour, or carob.

Have about three servings of legumes such as cooked beans and peas, skinless chicken, tofu, fish, shellfish, eggs, nuts, and lean red meats. (One serving is eight ounces of tofu, one cup of beans, or three ounces of fish or meat.) This gives you protein for the formation of various hormones, enzymes, nerve chemicals, and muscle tissue, and vitamin B12 and iron for red blood cell formation. (You can't really get these from tofu and beans.) Vitamin B6 is needed for the baby's nervous system and for protein metabolism.

Finally, have around eight glasses of fluid—fruit juice, green tea, or water. You need fluid to provide for the expanding blood volume that carries all the nutrients and oxygen you and your baby need.

Getting Those Extra 300 Calories

> Having to eat 300 extra calories a day sounds like a food lover's fantasy; but sad to say it isn't. (Eisenberg, Murkhoff, and Hathaway, *What to Expect When You're Expecting*, Workman, 1996, p. 85)

Use the first trimester to make sure you are eating enough calories for you and getting all your nutrients. Many nonpregnant women don't actually eat the so called 2,200 calories a day that research suggests the average woman should, so you may still need to increase your food intake in the first three months. When you enter your second trimester, metabolism speeds up and you need to increase your food intake by 300 calories.

Remember, 300 calories is only a couple of peanut butter sandwiches or a few glasses of milk. Think about how very tiny your baby-to-be is at the moment. An additional 300 calories is all the developing fetus needs to grow and thrive. If you are making sure you get enough protein, calcium, and iron, you will probably have already increased your calorie requirement significantly. So instead of eating that extra scoop of ice cream, you'll probably have to cut out sweets and fatty food and concentrate on lower-calorie, more nutritious food choices, like fruit and vegetable snacks.

If you are seriously over- or underweight, carrying more than one baby, or still in your teens, the 300 extra calorie rule may not apply. Very heavy or very thin women need to adjust their calorie intake appropriately. If you are carrying more fetuses, you need to add 300 calories for each baby, and if you are still growing yourself, you have special nutritional needs. In all these exceptions to the rule, you need to talk to your doctor.

To Supplement or Not to Supplement

If you were eating a normal balanced diet with adequate nutrients for several months prior to pregnancy, you should have adequate stores of the nutrients you need for pregnancy. If, however, you are like the great majority of women and your diet has been poor, taking a vitamin and mineral supplement is a good idea, especially if you smoked or drank, as these rob the body of nutrients. (I am using the past tense here, as I assume that now you are pregnant you have stopped smoking and drinking to excess in the interests of your baby-to-be. Cigarettes can seriously harm your baby, and studies have shown that so can too much alcohol.)

It's easy to become deficient in the nutrients the body needs most for pregnancy—vitamins C and D, iron, and folic acid—so doctors will routinely prescribe dietary supplements as soon as you become pregnant. There is still controversy about whether they are actually necessary. Research has not actually found any evidence that they should be used. According to some experts, "Vitamin supplements are rarely required during pregnancy provided a normal, balanced diet is followed." (Stavia Blunt, *Shaping Up*, Summersdale, 1997, p. 57) This may be true, but many of the new moms I talked to confessed that their diet prepregnancy was far from normal and balanced. Until they got pregnant most of them had never really thought that much about food, cooking, and shopping healthfully before.

Unless you have first-class knowledge of nutrition and are confident that you are eating a healthy diet, taking dietary supplements is advisable. The best way to make sure you are getting enough folic acid and iron, especially, is to take a supplement.

Warning one: Never take any kind of dietary supplement without consulting your doctor. An overdose of certain vitamins and minerals—vitamins A and D, for example—when you are pregnant could hurt you and your baby-to-be. Talk to your doctor about prenatal vitamins and which ones you should take, and you will be given a prescription. Self-prescription can be dangerous. Critics warn that high doses of certain vitamins can be harmful. Here's what you need to know about the potential hazards of supplements:

Vitamin A—High doses of beta carotene (the plant form of vitamin A) over long periods can turn skin orange. High doses can also be toxic with symptoms such as nausea, headache, and blurred vision.

Vitamin B3—High doses cause temporary flushing like a hot flash. Very high doses may cause abnormalities in liver function.

Vitamin D—At high doses, possible problems include nausea, headache, diarrhea, loss of appetite, and dangerously high levels of calcium in the blood.

Vitamin E—At large doses, nausea, diarrhea, headache, fainting, and heart palpitations are possible.

Zinc—Large doses may cause nausea and vomiting.

Iron—High iron levels may increase the risk of heart disease.

If you do take a supplement check that your supplements have the following:

- No more than 800 micrograms RE of vitamin A
- No more than 10 micrograms of vitamin D
- No more than 250 milligrams of calcium and 25 milligrams of magnesium if you are taking iron; these interfere with iron absorption (remember, 1,250 is the recommended calcium requirement)
- 200 to 300 milligrams of calcium
- 400 micrograms of folic acid
- The recommended daily allowance of vitamins C and B
- The recommended daily allowance of iron and zinc; lack of zinc, manganese, and amino acid imbalances have been linked to fetal abnormalities

- Avoid aspirin preparations. Aspirin has been linked to fetal abnormalities, bleeding, and complications during delivery. Supplements and sweeteners containing the amino acid phenylalanine can harm your baby, too.
- This is so important I'll repeat it. *All women of childbearing age should make sure their daily diet includes sufficient folic acid requirements for a pregnant woman.* Folic acid deficiency is linked to birth defects. This B vitamin must be present in the body in the six weeks following conception. Since most women do not know they have conceived until several weeks after, it is important to have an adequate supply of this vitamin at all times.
- If you want to take herbs during pregnancy, again make sure you consult with an expert. Alfalfa is a good source of vitamins and minerals, especially vitamin K, which is essential for blood clotting. St. John's wort and shepherd's purse help uterine contractions at birth. Burdock root, dandelion, ginger, and nettle help enrich your milk. Blessed thistle, blue cohosh, and squaw vine are beneficial in the last month of pregnancy, but do not take at any other time. Red raspberry leaf tea is also beneficial for uterine contractions and for enriching milk.

Avoid these herbs when you are pregnant: angelica, barberry, black cohosh, bloodroot, cat's claw, celandine, cottonwood bark, dong quai, feverfew, goldenseal, lobelia, Oregon grape, pennyroyal, rue, and tansey.

> *Warning two:* "Vitamin Pills are not a substitute for a good balanced diet" (Connie Marshall, *From Here to Maternity*, Conmar, 1994, p. 27) and "No pill, however complete, can replace a good diet" (Eisenberg, Murkoff, and Hathaway, *What to Expect When You're Expecting*, Workman, 1996, p. 89).

Don't think because you are taking a pill every day, it doesn't matter anymore what you eat or don't eat. It just doesn't work that way. The best way to get vitamins and minerals into your body and to your baby-to-be is through the food you eat. They can be utilized most effectively when ingested in this natural way. And pills don't give you energy, fiber, and water, either.

You may find that taking the supplements every day makes you feel sick. If that's the case, it might be best to take them last thing at night. They may be impossible to take some days when you are suffering from morning sickness. Try to take them when you can. Don't fret about the odd missed day, but do remember that it is during the first trimester that the development of fetal abnormalities is most likely to occur in cases of vitamin and mineral deficiency.

Weighing In

Concentrate on nutrients and not calories during pregnancy. Try to eat sensibly and healthily. Let your weight be the guide for how well you are doing. Once a week you should weigh yourself. Try to keep to the same day and time of day when you weigh yourself and use a scale that is reliable. Weighing yourself naked is best, too, as your clothing does represent some weight.

In the first trimester your weight shouldn't fluctuate too much. In the second and third trimester you should see a weight gain of about a pound or so a week. If that's not happening, eat more nutritious foods. If you are gaining more than a pound or so a week, adjust your diet— but don't cut out the nutrients you need.

8

Problems with Food

"I felt so sick during my pregnancy. I thought I would never enjoy food again."

"I was never a big eater, but when I got pregnant I was ravenous 24 hours a day."

"The worst part for me was getting constipated all the time. It made me feel so heavy."

"It was so depressing. I got gestational diabetes. I couldn't even eat what I wanted when I got pregnant."

It's bad enough losing your waistline and seeing your body shape change when you get pregnant. It's darn right unfair that we also often encounter an assortment of problems with food and digestion that not only take the enjoyment out of eating, but can make us feel tired, irritable, and unhappy with how we look.

Morning Sickness

About half of us will experience nausea and vomiting in the first trimester. This can leave you looking pale and tired. Also remember, it may be called morning sickness, but that doesn't mean it only happens first thing in the morning. It can strike any time of day.

There does not seem to be any cure for nausea that works for everyone. Antinausea drugs are off limits during pregnancy, but there are ways you can help yourself. Common remedies include vitamin B supplements. Some women find relief by wearing bands around their wrists that put pressure on the inner wrist. This type of acupressure may reduce the sensation of nausea. You can get them at your local drug store.

If your nausea and vomiting are not too severe, you can usually deal with them by following a few simple rules (if it is severe, consult your doctor):

- Before you go to bed, have a protein or complex carbohydrate snack to help prevent low blood sugar in the morning, which causes nausea.
- A diet high in protein and complex carbohydrates will help fight nausea. Good nutrition will, too.
- Drink plenty of fluids. Vomiting makes you dehydrated.
- Keep your mouth fresh and clean. This will reduce nausea and decrease the risk of damage to your teeth and gums.
- If you wake up in the night hungry, eat a few crackers. You might want to keep them by your bed!
- Eat plain, simple food. Avoid spices and junk food.
- Eat small amounts, often.
- Do not go without food or drink because of the nausea. You will feel worse.
- Herbs such as ginger, taken in capsule or tea form, can help combat nausea, as can raspberry leaf tea, peppermint, and dandelion. Known for its stomach-soothing powers, ginger tea is a tasty, soothing remedy for mild nausea. Use two teaspoons of powdered ginger per cup of boiling water and steep for ten minutes. Add honey or lemon for extra flavor.
- Try hydrotherapy treatment. Dip a towel in comfortably hot water and wring it out. Place it over your midriff from armpits to hips for a good fifteen minutes with a hot water bottle on your abdomen.
- Make sure you take a prenatal vitamin supplement to make up for the nutrients you might not be getting.
- Minimize stress. Morning sickness is more common among women who have a lot of stress in their lives.
- Make sure you get plenty of rest. Fatigue can make nausea worse.

Typically, morning sickness confines itself to the first three months of pregnancy. It can go on longer than that, though, and throughout your pregnancy you may experience the odd bout of nausea. You need to be concerned only if nausea and vomiting are interfering with healthy weight gain. If this is the case, hospitalization may be necessary to ensure that your baby gets adequate nutrition.

Morning sickness may prevent you from gaining any weight at all in the first trimester. Some women even lose weight. There is no cause for alarm; you can make up for this in the second trimester when food tastes good again. If it interferes with your weight gain in the second trimester, it is important that you consult your doctor.

Pregnancy Myth: Girls make you sick

"I really thought that I was going to have a boy when I found out I was pregnant. Then morning sickness struck. I was sick 24 hours a day from week 6 to 18. Everyone insisted that I was having a girl. I had a girl."

I suffered from bad morning sickness and had a boy, and many mothers say they were sick for both their boys and their girls. But there could be a grain of truth in this pregnancy myth. Research does indicate that increased sickness may mean that you are having a girl. Morning sickness tends to be associated with high levels of the hormone HCG, and girls often have higher HCG levels. HCG is the hormone that is thought to be partly responsible for triggering zones in the brain connected with nausea.

Constipation

There's nothing worse than that blocked-up feeling when you are constipated. Throughout my pregnancy I suffered from problems with constipation. It made me feel heavy, tired, and listless. I hated the thought of all that food and those toxins just sitting there.

Most of us feel better when we have regular bowel movements. We feel lighter, fresher, and more energetic. Constipation makes us feel bloated and out of sorts. It slows our metabolism, too. During pregnancy, when you feel tired and heavy already, constipation can be make you feel even heavier. Difficulty passing stools is a common problem during pregnancy. Hormonal changes, functional changes in the intestine, and pressure on the lower bowel and rectum all make constipation likely to occur. The iron in your prenatal vitamins may also be making your stools hard and black. If the problem persists, you may have to think about other ways to get enough iron.

If you are reading this and you never have problems with constipation, that's great. Your system has adapted quickly to your pregnancy. Chances are you have a great diet, too. You only need to be concerned if you get diarrhea. Consult your doctor if this is the case.

If you do suffer from constipation, there are ways you can fight back.

- Make sure you eat enough fiber. Add a couple of tablespoons of bran to a high-fiber breakfast cereal. Don't go wild, though, as bran moves quickly through your system and could rob your body of nutrients. Eat lots of fresh fruit and vegetables. Avoid food that constipates and is high in fat and sugar. Avoid convenience foods.
- Drink lots and lots of liquids and unsweetened juices—hot water with lemon or prune juice.
- Get moving. Exercise may loosen things.
- If constipation is bad, this can lead to hemorrhoids, internal or external, and they are very painful. You may have burning, itchy sensations or even bleeding when you try to have a bowel movement. If you get hemorrhoids, try to avoid sitting or standing too long in one place. Treat with warm soaks and anesthetic sprays. Cold witch hazel can help shrink hemorrhoids. Walk at least a mile a day and increase the amount of roughage and water.

If these don't work, see your doctor. You may need to be prescribed a stool softener. Try to avoid the use of laxatives when you are pregnant. They are too harsh for your system right now. They can also make you reliant on them.

Gas

Some days you might feel as if you are going to explode. Gas, like other digestive upsets, is a common complaint during pregnancy. Even foods that don't usually make you gassy will now. You can alleviate the problem by keeping a food diary to determine what is causing the gas. Avoiding big meals and eating little and often will also help. Be sure you do not overcook vegetables, and do eat more fresh fruit and vegetables.

Gestational Diabetes

Pregnancy hormones cause blood glucose levels to rise. For some of us, the pancreas just can't keep up with the demands for the extra insulin to keep blood sugar levels in balance. Gestational diabetes affects about 4 percent of pregnant women who have never had any symptoms of diabetes before. It usually happens sometime after the twentieth week.

If you get diabetes during pregnancy, you increase your chances of having a larger baby. The extra glucose circulating in your system crosses the placenta to the fetus, which then starts making its own insulin. With too much glucose and insulin, the baby-to-be puts on more weight than usual. Insulin is the hormone that helps you convert food to energy. If there are problems with insulin, then even if you have a lot of sugar in your system you can't utilize it effectively.

Most doctors will screen for diabetes at around twenty-four weeks of pregnancy. Screening includes being given a high sugar drink, and a blood sample will be taken a few hours later. Once the condition is detected, it can be managed and potential problems avoided.

Treatment will involve a change in diet. Your doctor will prescribe one recommended by the American Diabetes Association. This diet will help you control your blood sugar levels. An exercise routine will also be advised. If the problem can't be managed with diet and exercise alone, you may need insulin.

If you get gestational diabetes, it is very important to follow your prescribed diet and exercise plan. Be comforted by the knowledge that the condition is temporary. With just a little discipline on your part you can make sure that your baby-to-be is healthy and you are, too.

After delivery, your metabolism will usually return to normal. Don't relax too much about diet and exercise, though. If you have had gestational diabetes, you could be at increased risk of getting full-blown diabetes later in life. For your own sake and the sake of your family, stick to a healthy exercise and eating plan that will minimize your chances of getting diabetes. Weight management is crucial, as there is a close link between diabetes and obesity.

Disordered Eating Habits

We've already covered this in Part One, Chapter Five, but it bears repeating: If you have a history of dysfunctional eating, talk to your doctor. Eating disorders during pregnancy are dangerous. Your doctor may not know that much about the illness, so you may need to seek advice elsewhere in your community. Call your local hospital and ask for information about treatment and support groups or contact the addresses listed in the resource section of this book. There is help out there.

Bed Rest

If you have a high-risk pregnancy or are not gaining sufficient weight and bed rest is advised, it will affect your eating habits. Weeks or even months in bed can seem like a life sentence. Overeating out of boredom is understandable, but it is more important than ever that you pay attention to excellent nutrition to maximize your chances of delivering a healthy baby. Try to see the positive, and use your time to do all those things you wanted to but never had the time. Read novels. Write in your journal. If you can sit up, use a laptop and surf the Net. Talk to friends and family on the phone. Learn a language. Study. Use audio tapes if you find reading too tiring. Knit. Sew. Draw. Meditate. Relax.

I'm So Hungry

Pregnancy is a time for extremes. You have never been so big. You have never felt so happy. You have never felt so anxious. You have never felt so tired. You have never felt so sick. You have never felt so hungry.

Even if you are carefully watching your weight and eating a healthy diet, there will be times when every pregnant woman feels an uncontrollable urge to eat. You need to eat. You need to eat now. Never stand between a pregnant woman and food. You might also get strange food cravings that can interfere with your diet plans. Until the craving is satisfied, you feel empty inside. The hunger won't go away. Nutritionists don't really know why, but there are definite taste changes in pregnancy. You may go completely off tea or coffee, for example, and crave foods you never really liked before. Some women even crave nonfoods like coal! This could be explained by the body trying to get some of the minerals it needs. Do not give in to the non-food cravings, since your body can't absorb them properly.

When ravenous hunger or a bizarre food craving strikes, you may feel out of control. It is during these times that poor food choices are often made. Everywhere you go you will encounter a ready supply of ready-to-eat, nutritionally disastrous food. It's so easy to succumb!

Making sure you don't get too hungry by eating every two to three hours will help, but one way to cope when these sudden urges strike is to carry with you a supply of food that is healthy and won't make the weight pile on. Just a little forethought is required. Try to surround yourself with healthy snacks like these:

Health food bars
Apples
Bananas
Crackers and cheese
Grapes
Dried fruit
Carrots
Whole-wheat pretzels
Low-fat cereal

Yes, I know—it's not quite the same as a double chocolate cookie. But in time you may really begin to enjoy these alternative snacks. It's amazing how your taste buds adapt. Ask anyone who used to drink sugar in their coffee or tea and has given it up. Now they just can't stand having sugar in their drinks.

If you do use dietary common sense and make healthier food choices, you may surprise yourself and discover that you don't want to eat unhealthily anymore because healthy tastes better. Not only is it great for the health of your baby-to-be, but it makes you look and feel better, too.

Rare is the woman who does not experience some kind of problem with food and eating when she is pregnant. There are ways you can help yourself feel better, but if at times you get despondent, remember that in most cases the problems are temporary. They usually disappear when you have given birth.

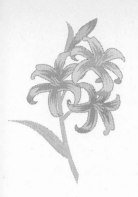

9

Exercise?

IN THE POPULAR AND VERY FUNNY *GIRLFRIENDS' GUIDE TO PREGNANCY Diary* (Pocket, 1996) Vicki Iovine lists the top ten reasons not to exercise. With reasons from "you will gain weight anyway" to "you are just too tired," Iovine has a point. Being pregnant is hard enough work anyway. It's tempting to forget about exercise for the whole nine months. Iovine assumes, though, that most of us hate to exercise, pregnant or not, in the first place. Even though some of us do hate exercise, there are some of us who actually enjoy it. And even if we don't really like it, we make the decision to exercise because we know it is good for us. It keeps our muscles and bones strong. It keeps our heart strong, too. It stimulates our metabolism so we burn calories faster. It makes us feel and look good. It gives us greater confidence about our bodies.

Is Exercise Safe During Pregnancy?

Exercise is an important part of my life, so when I first became pregnant, I read all I could find on pregnancy. I learned that most older research on exercise during pregnancy had been done on animals and is of questionable merit. More recent research on how the fetus adapts to exercise is illuminating. Athletes and joggers and dancers were studied during their active pregnancies. The results showed that even though blood does shift away from the uterus during strenuous exercise, the baby-to-be isn't harmed. Fears about retardation, low birth weight, and spinal defects are also unfounded. The studies reveal, too, that contrary to popular belief, labor and delivery are not easier for athletes. However, some doctors feel fitness is a definite benefit when it comes to delivery. It helps women cope with the stresses of pregnancy better.

There is clearly no need to stop exercising when you are pregnant. Doctors agree that it is safe. In the words of Dr. Jacobs, "It is safe to exercise when you're pregnant. Non-weight-bearing exercise like swimming is great. As for more intense exercise, it is fine as long as your body is used to it. You can continue your current exercise program provided you make certain modifications. If you are an avid exerciser, make sure you keep your heart rate down. You are not exercising to sweat and lose weight, but to strengthen your body. There is no real proof that vigorous exercise produces smaller babies or increases the risk of preterm labor, but most doctors would recommend against it during pregnancy. The first trimester is the best time to exercise, but you'll probably feel too tired. In the second trimester you'll have more energy, but your body will slow you down. For all pregnant women, I recommend regular exercise. I'd only have reservations if a woman had never exercised before. She must start very gradually and slowly."

The Benefits of Exercise When Pregnant

Exercise during pregnancy has many benefits. It can lift your spirits and give you a sense of well being. It can be a great de-stressor. It may help you feel more energetic, and you may cope with labor and delivery better. Exercise can also relieve backache, help prevent constipation and varicose veins, and even alleviate morning sickness. It will help you maintain your cardiovascular fitness during pregnancy and strengthen your bones and muscles. It will also help you control your weight. Don't forget, too, that if you exercise, you can eat more.

If weight management is your goal, sensible exercise during pregnancy is a must. Exercise burns calories. Keeping active will help you control your weight. And it's not just the calories you burn during exercise. Studies have shown that exercise continues to stimulate your metabolism for several hours after exercise. You just burn calories more efficiently if you are fit.

Be Sensible

Before you rush to put another block on your step, or think about that marathon you want to run, you have to be sensible. You can't exercise in the same way anymore. You have a baby on board. Studies on exercise and pregnant women come up with the same findings. You can exercise, provided you are sensible. This applies even if you don't exercise but have an active daily life that involves a lot of standing, carrying, lifting, and so on.

Being sensible means listening to your body and paying attention to any signals it sends you—for example, pain or tiredness. Stop exercising immediately if you experience any of the following:

- Bleeding or spotting or heavy discharge. Consult your doctor.
- Pain of any sort. Experienced exercisers need to be most careful here. They are used to going for the burn and working through pain. Don't do this when you are pregnant. Consult your doctor if pain persists.
- Dizziness, faintness, fatigue, difficulty breathing, rapid heartbeat. Consult your doctor if symptoms persist.
- Contractions of any sort. Consult your doctor.
- A gush of fluid. In most cases this is probably urine, but it could be amniotic fluid. Consult your doctor.
- If any unusual symptoms occur during exercise or there are complications to your pregnancy, consult your doctor.

Here's a very brief summary of the American College of Obstetricians and Gynecologists Guidelines for exercising when pregnant (ACOG Technical Bulletin No. 189, February 1994):

1. You can exercise when you are pregnant, but keep it mild to moderate. Three times a week is recommended.
2. After the first trimester, don't lie flat on your back for toning or strengthening exercises.
3. Don't stand or sit in the same position for long periods of time for toning and strengthening exercises.
4. Modify your intensity when exercising aerobically. You'll have less oxygen circulating and will need to stop when tired. Never exercise to exhaustion, and avoid vigorous exercise.

Ensure that your heart rate does not exceed 140 beats per minute. (If you count about 50 beats in 20 seconds, you are doing OK. A good investment would be a watch that monitors your pulse when you are exercising.)

5. You can do weight-bearing exercises, but non-weight-bearing exercise such as cycling and swimming are best. They are easier to continue and carry less risk of injury.

6. Avoid any exercise that risks injury to your abdomen. Don't engage in activities that require jumping, jarring, or rapid changes of motion. Avoid hard surfaces when you exercise.

7. Avoid exercise that involves balance, especially in the third trimester.

8. Don't work out in too hot an environment. Stay cool when exercising and wear cool, loose clothing. Don't raise your temperature to higher than 100.4°F.

10. Drink lots of fluids and water before, during, and after exercise.

11. Ensure that you are eating enough calories to sustain you, your baby, and the exercise routine.

12. Precede exercise with a five-minute warmup such as slow walking, and gradually cool down after exercise. Finish your exercise with gentle stretching.

After pregnancy, build up gradually to your prepregnancy exercise routine.

How Much Exercise Should I Do, and for How Long?

How much exercise you do and what type is safe depends on your own fitness level. Studies have shown that walking, swimming, slow jogging, stationary biking, and low-impact aerobics are safe for periods ranging up to 45 minutes three times a week.

If you are very fit, you might find these guidelines too moderate. You will have to listen to your body and adjust accordingly. Common sense should tell you when it is time to modify your exercise routine. If you have exercised previously, continuing your exercise program is unlikely to be harmful, unless the exercise is too vigorous. If you have not exercised before, you need to be more careful and should consult with your doctor and increase your exercise intensity and frequency gradually. Strenuous activity should be avoided, especially in the first and last trimester. At other times it should never exceed fifteen minutes. "The safe and realistic goal of exercise during pregnancy is to maintain a reasonable level of fitness." (Connie Marshal, *From Here to Maternity*, Conmar, 1997, p. 30)

Being pregnant is no excuse to become a couch potato without guilt. Neither is it time to start training for a marathon. Moderation is the key. Aim to maintain your current fitness levels, not to increase them. Continue to do the activities you normally do, as long as you follow safety guidelines. Target heart rate has been the usual way to calculate how intense your exercise is. Your heartbeat shouldn't exceed 140 beats a minute. If you, like me, find it really hard to do all those pulse measuring calculations, there is a simpler way. You should be able to carry on a conversation when you are exercising. If you can't, or you find that you have to keep drawing huge breaths to speak, you are exercising too hard and you should stop or modify to a lower intensity. You need to aim for an intensity level that is halfway between very easy and very difficult.

We Are All Different

"I used to be fit before I got pregnant. I'm just in my second trimester, and even looking at my sneakers makes me feel exhausted."

"Running in the morning helped me cope with my morning sickness and headaches."

"I've never liked exercise. I'm certainly not going to start now I'm pregnant."

"I ran thirty to thirty-five miles a week before I got pregnant. When I got pregnant I still ran every day, but not for so far or for so long in the last few months. I had been for a run on the day I delivered."

"In my eighteenth week I had to stop exercising and go on bed rest for ten weeks. There were problems with my placenta. For an active person like me, it was a nightmare."

"I kept very active during my pregnancy, biking, swimming, or walking every day. I'm sure it helped me when I delivered."

Each of us will cope with and experience pregnancy in our unique way. And we will cope with the subject of activity during pregnancy in our own unique way, too. What one woman can do when pregnant, another may not be able to. Some can be very active; some can't. Some will exercise moderately. Some will have a strict fitness regime.

There is no one way to exercise during pregnancy. You have to find what works best for you. If you can run every day and you feel great, good for you. Just be sensible. If you are too exhausted to exercise, don't pressure yourself. Have a rest day. Perhaps you could try and do a little gentle walking tomorrow. It might make you feel better.

Just as with your healthy eating plan, common sense and moderation is required. Listen to your body and how it feels. Do what you can.

Exercise and Body Changes During Pregnancy

One of the first things you may notice when you exercise while pregnant is that you get out of breath quicker. With all that baby-to-be growing inside you, your lung capacity is reduced. You might at times feel like you are really breathing heavily. This is not unusual. Your body will soon learn to adapt. Difficulty with breathing will be more noticeable for weight-bearing activities such as running than for activities such as swimming, and it will also be more prominent during the last trimester.

Blood sugar levels can fall very rapidly when you're pregnant. Try to carry snacks with you, and to avoid fatigue, don't exercise on an empty stomach. As your pregnancy progresses you may find that you have less and less energy for exercise. You will need to modify your exercise program to accommodate declining exercise levels.

You might also find that you ache more after exercise. This is because lactic acid buildup increases, as your respiratory system is less efficient when you are pregnant. You can avoid this with gentle stretching before and after exercise. You'll be more prone to losing your balance and getting injuries, too, because pregnancy hormones relax your ligaments and joints. Lower back pain could occur, too. You have to cope with a shift in your center of gravity. So you need to be careful of activities that require balance and coordination.

None of these changes happen overnight, though. You won't suddenly have to deal with them all at once. They will appear gradually, and as they do you will learn to adapt on a daily basis. One change you might notice right away though is that you sweat a lot more when you exercise. Even when resting, a pregnant woman has a higher than normal basal metabolic rate. She will feel warmer. So when you start exercising, your body cools you down by sending all that blood to the skin surface to make you feel cooler. The fitter you are and the more efficient your cooling system is, the more you will tend to sweat.

Whatever level of fitness you are, you must beware of overheating. This is dangerous for you and baby-to-be. "The critical temperature is in excess of 100.4°F (38°C)" writes Joan Butler in *Fit and Pregnant* (Acorn, 1996, p. 43). Animal studies have shown that overheating can cause spinal defects in a fetus. Your baby can't cool off with sweating as you do. So be careful of hot baths and saunas and Jacuzzis, hot and humid weather, and high fevers and illness.

Dehydration and heat loss during exercise can occur more quickly during pregnancy and seriously alter fetal well-being. Excessive exertion can reduce blood, oxygen, and glucose supply from the uterus to your working muscles. It can also injure your spine. Make sure you drink before, during, and after exercise. Don't exercise strenuously for long periods of time. Be aware of your body temperature and avoid overheating.

If you are going to exercise regularly, you must eat more. Not only must you eat a healthy, balanced diet to fulfill the metabolic requirements of pregnancy, but you need also to eat enough to have the energy to exercise. If you are gaining weight at a steady rate, it is likely that you are getting enough calories for you, your baby-to-be, and your exercise. If you are not gaining steadily, cut down on the exercise a little and make sure you replace the nutrients you lose during exercise.

Finally, you may feel uncomfortable when you exercise because you have to pass water frequently. You may leak and be unable to control it. Don't worry—you are not incontinent. This happens when you are pregnant. You might find that exercise stimulates the need for bowel movements, too. Wear a large sanitary pad and make sure you exercise near restrooms.

If You're Still Concerned about Exercise

Although I knew exercise was safe during pregnancy, I still had concerns: The image of my baby-to-be bumping around in the womb when I jogged haunted me. Was I hurting him? I discovered that I was worrying needlessly—the fetus is well cushioned in the womb. He may even enjoy the gentle bouncing sensation of exercise!

I worried that the blood flow shifting to my working muscles when I exercised would harm my baby-to-be. Again I was worrying needlessly—the only way I could have harmed my baby-to-be would have been if I had exercised vigorously and intensely for long periods of time. Blood continues to flow to the fetus when exercise is moderate. If exercise gets too hard, though, diversion of blood to the uterus is probably lessened and fetal heartbeat lowered.

Another concern was that exercise would make my baby-to-be smaller. I found out that there is no conclusive evidence to suggest that this is the case.

I was afraid, too, that I might miscarry or have premature labor. Early in my first trimester I came back from a jog and noticed a brown and red discharge. I immediately called my doctor in panic. After an examination he said that there was nothing wrong. I asked him if I should continue jogging. Would it make me likely to miscarry? Dr. Douglas's answer reassured me: "You can play it safe and go on bed rest, but in my experience if you are going to miscarry in the first trimester you will whether you jog or not. Just be sensible with your exercise and don't overdo it."

There is absolutely no evidence that moderate, sensible exercise will increase the likelihood of miscarriage or problems with your pregnancy. Forget all those Hollywood films you have seen with the heroine collapsing as soon as she gets a little active. To repeat, you only put your pregnancy in danger if activity is exhausting, strenuous, and violent—not if it is moderate. "In fact, moderate activity in healthy, well-nourished pregnant women can actually prevent some health problems like excessive weight gain, poor posture and lower back pain, fatigue and poor body image" (Joan Marie Butler, *Fit Pregnancy*, Acorn, 1996, p. 45)

Types of Exercise Most Suitable for Pregnancy

Swimming is the number one doctor-recommended exercise during pregnancy. You can work on your cardiovascular fitness and not worry about getting injuries. You can rest and float when you want to. You can swim from conception to the day of your delivery. You can practice your breathing, and you are less likely to overheat in the pool.

Walking is another highly recommended exercise routine during pregnancy. It is low-impact, gentle on your body, and won't damage your joints. It's a great alternative to running and if done properly with correct form and purpose, it can be as invigorating as running. Walking is good for relieving stress. Make sure you empty your bladder before you go out, though, and avoid walking in very hot, humid weather. Walking is also a good time for you to work on your posture.

Biking is also good to do when you are pregnant. A stationary bike is perhaps the safest, as you won't be able to fall and injure yourself. Avoid getting your heart rate over 140 beats per minute. Biking does not strain your joints and ligaments, but still gives you aerobic fitness. Make sure your bike fits you and is comfortable to use. As your pregnancy progresses, you may have to alter your biking position.

If you do aerobics, you may find as your pregnancy progresses that it is harder and harder to keep up. Your changing body requires that you modify some of the exercises to avoid injury or discomfort. Don't do any abdominals after the fourth month. Make sure your teacher is qualified to teach pregnant women, and watch that heartbeat. Low-impact aerobics is best. Make sure also you follow the exercise guidelines during pregnancy mentioned earlier. You might find a prenatal exercise class, which is also great for meeting other pregnant women and making friends.

Weight training is a great complement to the aerobic exercise listed above. It strengthens and tones your muscles, which is especially important during pregnancy. You will soon find out when baby-to-be is born how much you need strong arm and back muscles. Weight training is fine, but use light to moderate weights. Don't do exercises that stress your lower back or abdominal muscles. Make sure you breathe properly and warm up before and cool down afterwards.

As your body changes, so must your weight training or toning program. Remember, you are conditioning not to reshape your body, but to retain tone and fitness.

Make sure you stretch, warm up, and cool down before and after exercise. If you don't, you risk injury. A warmup can be as simple as walking easily before you start pacing, or doing some easy laps in the pool before you swim with purpose. Follow warming up with stretching. Gently stretch the major muscles you will be working in your workout. For example, with running you would stretch your calf, hamstrings, and quads before you run. Cool down at the end of your workout. This lowers your heartbeat gradually and reduces muscle soreness. Do some easy laps again, for example. Then finish with more stretching.

Now that you are pregnant, it's more important than ever to not skip warmup, cool-down, and stretching. It helps your body adjust to the demands of exercise and relaxes and prepares you. It also avoids the risk of injury. It is time well spent.

If you loathe the gym there are alternative ways to strengthen and tone your body. Try yoga or Tai Chi.

Avoid any sport that could injure your belly in any way. Avoid games with balls like football or tennis or hockey. Avoid boxing and fencing. Avoid gymnastics and ice-skating because of the danger of falls. Avoid diving. Avoid rock climbing. Avoid in-line skates. Avoid skiing and water sports. Other activities such as hiking, rowing, and canoeing and winter sports should only be engaged in if you are well experienced in them before and modify your program accordingly.

Jogging is usually fine to continue during pregnancy, provided you are used to it and don't turn jogging into sprinting. In general it is safe as long as you modify. If you have never run before, now is not the time to start. Proper warmup and cool-down, as well as stretching before and after you jog, are important. Make sure you jog in an area that is safe and that is near a restroom! Later in your pregnancy you may find jogging strains your joints too much as you gain weight. You'll probably want to combine jogging with walking.

For Those Who Don't Exercise

If you exercise moderately during your pregnancy, there are many health benefits. Because you will be burning more calories, you won't be gaining too much weight. If this still hasn't motivated you to join a gym or start an exercise routine, try to get exercise into your life somehow. There are many ways you can do this. Walk just a little more each day. Don't park quite so near the stores. Keep active. Dance to some music you love. Avoid sitting for too long. Take the stairs, not the elevator, and be more active in your daily life.

Exercise Tips

Try to make fitness a welcome part of life, not a chore. Think of it as time when you can do something positive for yourself and for baby. Be realistic, though, and don't overdo it. Rest when you are tired. You are pregnant. You won't be able to compete in the Olympics this year. Aim to do some kind of aerobic activity three times a week for about 45 minutes. This will boost your metabolism so you burn calories quicker. It will also give you a feeling of well-being. Remember, too, that muscles burn more calories than fat does. So make sure you do some strengthening and toning of your muscles.

Include variety in your exercise. That way you won't get bored. It will also stop you from overworking the same muscles and joints. Stay hydrated. Drink water before, during, and after exercise. Pay attention to your posture when you exercise, and make fitness fun. It really can be. Use it as a time to collect your thoughts about baby-to-be, too. Daydream about what he or she will look like. What kind of a mother you will be.

There is no published evidence to support the belief that the fitter you are, the easier your delivery, but many of the doctors I talked to said that fitness was a definite plus when it came to labor and delivery. Deliveries were no faster or less painful, but the fitter women coped better with the ordeal. Here's what some women thought about their fitness levels and how it affected their pregnancy and delivery.

"I really felt that because I exercised daily when I was pregnant I was stronger in the delivery room. I breathed well and I had the energy to keep going for nearly 39 hours, 10 of which were hard labor."

"Exercise during pregnancy gave me confidence about delivery. I wasn't worried at all. I knew I could cope."

"I think being in shape definitely made my labor and delivery easier."

"I don't think exercise helped me in labor and delivery, but it definitely helped me during my pregnancy."

"The only way I could stop feeling so sick in the early months was by going for a run."

"Whenever I felt really horrible, exercise always lifted my spirits."

"I was too tired to exercise during pregnancy, but my daily walks really helped energize me."

Think of these nine months as a training period. You are in training to have a baby! You and your body need to work together so that when you have your baby-to-be, you won't be out of condition and listless, but energetic and fit to be a mom.

10

Healthy Tips for Your Blossoming Body

GAINING WEIGHT WHEN YOU ARE PREGNANT IS, ON THE ONE HAND, THE most natural thing in the world. But combined with an increased blood volume and an expanding uterus, weight gain brings with it a variety of potential problems. What's more, the weight gain takes place in a very short period of time, around six months, and your body is not given the chance to slowly adapt.

"Most of the problems that occur during pregnancy are the result of hormonal changes within the body, nutritional deficiencies or the shift in weight distribution caused by sudden weight gain." (James and Phyllis Balch, *Nutritional Healing*, Avery, 1997, p. 435) Here are some healthy tips to ease the discomforts caused directly by the increase in your weight in the months your body blossoms:

Backache

You won't gain weight in your back, but you may feel pain in your back because of the weight gain. Your added frontal weight can pull your lower spine out of alignment, and your expanding uterus will put pressure on ligaments in your lower back. These bodily changes make "backache one of the most usual complaints of pregnancy" (Dr. Jacobs). The more weight you gain, the worse the problem can be. It can get so bad that you might have to wear a maternity belt to support you when you walk. Here are a few things that may help alleviate backache:

- Try to keep weight gain within the required range
- Learn proper body mechanics. Lift things properly. Bend at the knees and not at the waist. Spread your feet apart with one slightly in front of the other. Lift objects to waist height only and don't lift heavy loads at all.
- When you get up from a lying position, roll to your side and lever your upper body with your arms to help you get up.
- When you sit, try and put your feet up and make sure your back is aligned. A little cushion to support your lower back might help, too.
- Avoid crossing your legs as this can promote circulation problems.

Sitting or standing for long periods of time can weaken your back, as can high-heeled shoes. Wear comfortable flat or low-heeled ones. Good posture is essential. You probably tend to lean back a little when you walk. Most pregnant women do. Trying to tilt the pelvis forward a little will help. To check your posture, stand with your back against a wall. Relax your knees and place your feet slightly apart. Press your shoulders against a wall and feel your spine elongating. If you have been walking with poor posture, you will feel the difference. Checking your posture when sitting is important, too. Choose a chair with a firm back and avoid slumping. When you go to sleep, lie on your side in the same position your baby-to-be lies in with knees drawn up. Later in your pregnancy, a pillow between your legs will help, too.

Include some gentle stretching and back strengthening exercises in your daily routine. When back pain strikes, this simple stretch might help:

Sit in a chair and lean your head down to your knees. Slowly uncurl one vertebra at a time until you are fully stretched up. This really feels good for the whole back. For the upper back, try shoulder and neck shrugs and circles. For the lower back, try pelvic rolls.

To strengthen your back try some gentle squats holding on to a chair.

Edema (Swollen Feet and Ankles)

Most women get some kind of swelling when they are pregnant, especially at the end of the day or when it is hot. It's a sign of a normal pregnancy and connected with the rise in estrogen levels and weight gain. Consult your doctor if swelling is rapid and sudden.

During pregnancy, certain hormones are produced that blunt your kidneys' ability to get rid of fluid. Fluids tend to build up in the bloodstream and then spill into your tissues. The problem is worse at the end of the day because gravity has pulled the fluid down. When you lie down at night, the fluid redistributes itself. The wide swings that occur in your weight, particularly in the third trimester, are due to sudden retention or release of this body fluid. Weight gain due to fluid retention will not stay with you or add to your permanent weight. Amazingly, by just two weeks postpartum your blood and fluid levels should be back to normal.

Here are a few tips to relieve the pain and discomfort of edema during pregnancy:

- Manage your weight gain. Excessive weight gain will put your legs under even more pressure.
- If you can, walk at least a mile a day. This helps keep the condition under control.
- Avoid diuretics as they can cause a serious imbalance in your body, and restrictive clothing, which can impede circulation.
- Don't restrict your fluid intake. Make sure you drink enough fluid to keep the kidneys working efficiently.
- Elevate your legs whenever you can.
- When you can, lie on your left side for twenty minutes or so during the day. Lying on your left side is recommended because it allows maximum flow of nutrients and blood to the placenta, which in turn helps your body absorb excess fluid.

Watch your diet. Salt plays a role in fluid retention. There was a time when doctors severely restricted the salt intake of a pregnant woman because they thought it caused toxemia, which is fluid retention and high blood pressure. Doctors now know that salt does not cause these conditions, but it can contribute to their development if taken in excess—so salt your food lightly.

Soaking your legs regularly in hot and cold water, making sure the last soak is cold to improve circulation, may help. If you get swollen fingers and feet, soak your hands and feet in warm water and make sure you wear flat, comfortable, loose-fitting shoes. Take your rings off if you have to.

You could also get a puffy, filled-out face. Extra fluids and weight show there, too. Nasal tissues swell, too, during pregnancy which is why nosebleeds and stuffy noses are common in pregnancy. Vaseline may help you avoid nasal dryness. Using a humidifier might help, too. If you get a nose bleed, pinch your nostrils together for a few minutes. Keep sitting up. Don't lie down. Increasing your intake of foods rich in vitamin C and cutting back on dairy products might be beneficial.

Faintness and Dizziness

You will certainly suffer from faintness and dizziness if you are not gaining enough weight. You might also feel dizzy if you skip meals or go too long without food. Without a supply of nutrients, blood sugar levels fall. You will feel shaky and may get headaches, too. To minimize the possibility of feeling dizzy, avoid lying on your back after the fifth month. Sleep on your side. If left on your back you could faint and undergo a serious drop in blood pressure. So be careful. Try also not to stand in one spot for too long. Your expanding uterus will compress the major arteries and trap blood, making your blood pressure drop. And don't change positions quickly. Always go from lying to sitting to standing slowly. Take your time and focus on what you are doing.

Fatigue

Gaining all that weight is tiring. Carrying it around is, too. Being pregnant is equivalent to tying six five-pound bags of salt or sugar or flour around your waist. You're going to get tired more quickly and out of breath.

Fatigue is not only due to weight gain. The demands of the fetus and tremendous hormone changes make you tired in the early months. Usually this wears off by the fifth month. Fatigue after that is more likely to be due to your weight gain. To cope with fatigue, try to create a balance between work and rest. Listen to your body. Rest when you have to. Don't do too much, and eat a well-balanced diet.

Heartburn

Your uterus pushes your stomach upwards as it grows. Pregnancy hormones slow digestion. Stomach acid can shoot back into your throat. It tastes disgusting and acid. At times, it can even hurt.

Once your baby-to-be is born, you should be free of heartburn. But for now, to relieve the condition take antacids recommended by your doctor. Try to sleep with your head elevated. Avoid spicy foods, which encourage the production of stomach acid, and eat small and frequent meals so your stomach does not get too full. Good posture will prevent further pressure on your stomach. Don't exercise right after a meal. Don't lie down after eating. You will see it all again!

Insomnia

As your body gets bigger and bigger, finding a comfortable position becomes challenging. Lying on your stomach and back is impossible. So you have to lie on your side. Lying on your left side seems to be the best sleeping position because it helps with problems of water retention. A cushion between your legs may help. A warm bath or foot massage might also relax you before you go to sleep. Don't take sleeping medications because, like all medications, your unborn baby takes them with you. Try a glass of warm milk and a cracker before you go to bed. Don't force yourself to sleep when you really can't. Read or do nonstrenuous chores until you are sleepy. Eating more food rich in the B vitamins might also help.

If you start to get dark circles under your eyes due to lack of sleep, you might want to camouflage with a beige cover stick. White makes you look more puffy. Applying a rose or peach blush in an upward sweep from cheekbone to temple can also help disguise fatigue.

Cramps

Posture altered by pregnancy may contribute to leg cramps. The forward shift of your weight strains your legs. It is also thought that cramping has to do with some problem with how your body absorbs calcium. So try to keep to a healthy diet and make sure you get your calcium. Milk is a good source of calcium, but some doctors believe it is associated with leg cramps because milk is high in phosphorus, which can interfere with calcium absorption. You might want to try and get your calcium from other sources. You can increase your calcium and potassium intake by eating foods such as almonds, bananas, grapefruit, low-fat cottage cheese, oranges, salmon, and low-fat yogurt.

Try sleeping with your legs elevated. Don't stand in one position too long during the day. Walk at least a mile a day if you can. When disaster strikes, try to flex your feet at the ankles. Or get your partner to do it for you. This will really ease the pain. Applying pressure and heat to the cramping area also helps. A warm bath and calf stretch before your go to bed could prevent cramps from occurring at all.

Numbness in Arms and Legs

You try to get up and one of your legs or arms refuses to cooperate. It has fallen asleep. Again, this is caused by your altered posture and weight gain. When you finally get your limb to move, it will probably tingle for a while.

Managing your weight, regular stretching, getting up slowly, and avoiding sudden, jerky movements will help ease numbness.

Pain

To accommodate your growing baby-to-be, your body has to make certain adjustments. You may feel pain when you walk due to increased movement in your hip, groin, and tailbone areas when you walk. There isn't much you can do except rest a lot and elevate your feet when you can. Near the end of your pregnancy you could get sore ribs when the uterus pushes against your rib cage. This will go away as soon as you have the baby. Practicing good posture, stretching your arms over your head, and changing positions frequently may help. The added weight will also stress your ligaments that hold up the uterus. You will feel pain all around your belly on sporadic occasions, usually in the fifth and eighth month. Again, resting and stretching will help. You could also get shooting pains in your vagina occasionally due to uterine pressure on your nerves. The best you can do about this is get off your feet and relieve the pressure.

When pain strikes, breathe deeply and bend toward the point of pain in order to let the ligaments relax. Rest in bed on your side until the pain passes. If pain persists, you should consult your doctor.

Stretch Marks

After you have your baby, you could be left with slight gray lines where your skin stretched. Stretch marks are associated with rapid weight gain. Once they appear, they are permanent, but they will be less noticeable with time.

So far there is no cream that removes stretch marks, so save your money! Retin-A has shown some promise, but this is out of bounds for pregnant and nursing moms. Other commonly suggested remedies, such as vitamin E oil, cocoa butter, and essential oils, help some women, but there is no evidence to suggest that they work. Taking care of your skin, gaining weight slowly and gradually, and keeping with the recommended range of weight gain are the best ways to prevent stretch marks. Many women who have given birth told me that apprehension about stretch marks actually transformed into pride—a permanent reminder of how their body worked an amazing miracle and created new life.

Itchy Skin

Itchy skin eruptions are another common side effect of pregnancy. You could get itchy skin as it stretches to accommodate your baby. I scratched and scratched when I was pregnant and got nasty sores on my stomach that hurt. This is called prickly heat, an itchy red rash that usually appears in skin creases and occurs when heat-swollen skin blocks the escape of perspiration.

Bathing, without scrubbing, in lukewarm water with mild soap, blotting skin dry, and dusting lightly with talcum powder might help. Keep your skin as cool as you can, and wear clothes of fabric that let your skin breathe like cotton. Don't scratch, as I did. Try soothing creams or anesthetic lotions. Keep skin clean, and avoid using too many sprays and cosmetics.

Frequent Urination

Everything gets bigger in pregnancy except your bladder, which shrinks.

Your growing uterus puts pressure on your bladder. Pregnant women have to spend a lot of time in restrooms both day and night. Don't be tempted to drink less—it won't help. You should still drink at least eight glasses of water a day.

Varicose Veins

As you gain weight during pregnancy, you may get varicose veins. The distended veins result from the pressure of your growing uterus on blood vessels. Usually these disappear when you have your baby. You can alleviate the pressure of your uterus on your legs by not sitting or standing for too long and resting with your feet up when you can. Aerobic exercise will also help improve circulation in the pelvic region and legs. Supportive hose might relieve discomfort, too. Don't wear elastic-topped knee socks, garters, belts, or high-heeled shoes.

Your Breasts

Your breasts go through a lot when you are pregnant. They increase in size by a couple of pounds. They become sore and tender, they may leak, and they get fuller and heavier in preparation for breastfeeding.

A warm washcloth should help soothe painful breasts. A good supportive bra is essential. Buy new bras that fit well. You may find that you increase a cup size or two. Mammary massage can also relieve soreness. Rub some massage oil or cream in your hands to warm it, then make large circles around the outside of your breasts, avoiding the nipples. Then massage each breast separately for a few minutes with smaller circles. Place both hands flat on each side of the dark area surrounding the nipple and slide your hands away to the edge of your breast.

The Nursing Pad

Pregnancy weight gain is not all in the belly. Weight does not go straight there. It also goes to the place most of us hate for it to go—

the hips, bottom, and thighs. You can understand why your belly is growing, but why is your rear growing, too? The extra weight on your hips, thighs, and buttocks is a necessary part of being pregnant. "Women typically put on an extra seven pounds of fat during pregnancy, which some experts have dubbed the 'nursing pad'—fat stores that are used up in pregnancy. Extra weight tends to settle around the hips and thighs, says Dr. Cox, whether a woman is pregnant or not." (Sarah McCraw, *American Baby*, Feb. 1999, p. 51)

The best you can do about the extra pounds gained in your lower body is to keep your weight within the desired range for your height and build, eat healthily, and keep active.

Your Belly

In the ninth month you will have about six to eight pounds of baby and three or so pounds of placenta, amniotic fluid, and uterus. As the fetus grows it tilts forward onto your abdominal muscles. Looser joints will make you feel slightly unsteady on your hips as you walk. You may start losing your balance on occasion. Your coordination will suffer, too, as your added load will make you less nimble. Being pregnant means an expanding waistline that will at times throw you off balance. Managing your weight, avoiding activities that require a lot of balance, and being careful as you go about your daily business are the best ways to manage that uncoordinated feeling.

Your growing belly may affect you in every way. You may feel different because of it. You will move differently because of it. You may feel pain because of it. You may feel incredible joy because of it. Everywhere you go it will remain the main attraction, whether you like it or not. People won't look you in the eye anymore. Your doctor will run a tape measure over it. Your partner may talk to it. People will look at it. You will gaze at it. As your pregnancy nears its end, you may even begin to think it is beautiful. And when baby-to-be is born, amazingly enough, for a very short while, you might even miss it!

Feeling Fat

Pregnancy brings with it countless changes, not only on the outside, but on the inside, too.

If you feel ashamed of your pregnant body, chances are you probably weren't that comfortable with your body before pregnancy, either. To be disappointed with your looks is to be disappointed with yourself. Pregnancy offers a remarkable opportunity for change—to improve your body image and create a more positive self-image.

Try to spend some time reflecting on how wise your body is when you have a baby. How necessary gaining weight is. How perfect it is for the creation of new life. Try to separate thinness from attractiveness. Use it as an opportunity to reprogram your attitudes. Instead of feeling fat, concentrate on how feminine you are. How womanly you are when you have a baby.

You want the best for your baby-to-be. So when you start to feel anxious about your weight gain, take a moment to think. You are not a slave to your emotions. Just because you feel worried or unhappy does not mean you have to make a poor food choice or starve yourself. You are in control. You can use common sense. Even if you don't make the best food choice, try to make a reasonable one. Pretzels are better than chips, for example. Be good to yourself, just as you would be good to your baby.

The earlier in your pregnancy you can start thinking positively about the beauty and benefits of an expanding middle, the better. Remember you are nourishing your child inside your womb. You want to be a good role model. Now is the time to break negative thinking. Do you want your child to be obsessed with his or her appearance? Of course not. You want them to be happy and healthy. So don't communicate stress and a negative self-image to your baby-to-be. If you want your child to feel positive about his or her body, it starts with you.

Body Image Boosting Tips

A positive self-image isn't easy. But improving your self-image will help you cope with the many changes both physical and emotional, as well as nurture the special connection between you and baby-to-be. Here are some tips on how to get into a healthy frame of mind about weight gain during pregnancy.

Remember you are not fat—you are pregnant. There is a world of difference. If you feel ill, tired, or sick and don't have the energy you used to, there is nothing wrong with you. Your body is working incredibly hard. You just need to rest and take it easy. Understand what is going on in your body. Learn all you can about your changing body. Visit libraries and bookstores. Attend classes. Get some awareness of where and how the weight is being distributed and why. There is a reason for every pound gained. Respect the wisdom of your body.

Never again will your baby be a part of you as he is now. Cherish this special time. Don't obsess about your expanding waistline. Turn your thoughts to something that makes you feel happy. Your baby-to-be. Your glowing skin. Your shining hair. Your incredible breasts. Concentrate on what's going on inside, not outside. The creation of new life is a miracle. Talk to other pregnant women. They'll probably be feeling as insecure as you are. Have a good laugh together. Talk to your partner. If you are feeling negative about yourself, continued intimacy between you and your partner will make you feel special and loved. Ask for unconditional support. If anyone in your life makes unwelcome comments about your appearance, tell him or her you are very sensitive about how you look and need them to be understanding.

Cooperate with your body. Look after yourself. Eat healthily. Increase your intake of food rich in the B vitamins and iron, such as brown rice, eggs, whole-grain cereal, fish, green leafy vegetables, oats, soy products, and wheat germ. These foods have a beneficial effect and will stop you feeling so tired, irritable, and cranky about the bodily changes you are experiencing. Get fresh air and exercise. If the scales depress you, remember that you won't be pregnant forever. And besides, being pregnant is not unattractive. You'll be surprised. Men often find it very seductive. Other women can treat you with respect.

Be good to yourself. Take care of your appearance. Have fun wearing those leggings and comfortable long sweaters. Get your hair done. Spend time doing what you enjoy. Stop being negative. Don't think you will never get back to your prepregnancy weight. You can. You know that with sensible diet and exercise, you can lose weight. Whenever people ask you about your weight, just tell them you have gained a sufficient amount.

And when you feel conflict between your needs and the needs of the baby, don't panic. This is normal. This is what being a mom is all about.

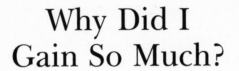

11

Why Did I Gain So Much?

AT THE ONSET OF PREGNANCY, TWENTY-FIVE TO THIRTY POUNDS SEEMS like a huge amount to gain. But by the time your due date draws near, you might find yourself with a weight gain in the range of forty to fifty pounds. Why did you gain so much?

Perhaps you ate too much.

"It was so hard to resist. When I started to show, everyone would encourage me to eat more. At restaurants even the waiters would urge me to have a dessert, saying 'Go on, you can.' I lost my will power completely."

The most likely cause of excessive weight gain during pregnancy is simple. You ate too much. After years of worrying about weight, getting pregnant seemed like a ticket to hog heaven. You could eat without guilt at last. Or perhaps you had morning sickness and couldn't get much down in the first trimester. In the second trimester you couldn't wait to make up for time lost. You found your taste buds again. No more nausea and gagging at the sight of food. Everything tasted delicious. You gained twenty-five pounds. During the third trimester you have a ferocious appetite. Your baby wants food. You eat and eat. Weight piles on.

Did you put on too much weight too soon?

"Before I was four months pregnant, I had already gained twenty pounds."

Overeating in the first few months is the most common weight management mistake moms make. In the first trimester you are only supposed to put on a few pounds. If you put on too much now, you will be stuck with the extra weight. This is because in the first trimester your calorie intake isn't shared by your baby, which is still an embryo. The placenta, which passes your nutrients on to the baby, isn't formed yet. And in the second and third trimesters, you can't really limit your weight gain too much, because it is now that your baby-to-be is really beginning to grow.

You don't actually need to eat much more than normal in the first trimester. In the second and third you will, but not now. Think how very tiny your baby is now and how minimal her caloric needs. You do, however, need to eat a healthy balanced diet appropriate for your age and build. Now is not the time to diet.

Perhaps you didn't eat much, but what you were eating was very fattening.

"I didn't think I ate too much. I had three good meals a day, but looking back it was all the chocolate, snacks, and chips in between that made me gain so much weight. I put on forty-nine pounds when I got pregnant. It was far too much."

Not only is how much you eat a contributory factor to weight problems during pregnancy, but what you eat. The quality of the food you eat that contributes to the weight gain is more important than the quantity.

Did you have a huge appetite?

"I just wanted to eat all the time. I couldn't stop, especially in my last trimester."

Almost every pregnant woman will notice that her appetite increases. You may even experience ravenous hunger and unusual food cravings. If you make wise and nutritious food choices, you can satisfy these cravings. However, if you eat junk food, you will still feel hungry. You'll need to eat more. You'll gain more weight.

Are you an emotional eater?

"I wanted my baby, but I was so scared about becoming a mom. I knew I'd have to give up a lot. I knew I'd have to grow up. After all, someone was going to rely on me now."

You may turn to food as comfort whenever you are worried, anxious, frustrated, angry, or indeed whenever you feel any kind of powerful emotion. Pregnancy is a time when many women experience a wide variety of emotions, some of them positive, but some of them distressing, too. You may be worried about coping, how a baby will change your life, how it will change your relationship with your partner, how it will affect your career, whether this is the right time to have a baby, whether you are responsible enough, and so on. Often, finding out what the underlying causes of your negative eating patterns are is the first step on the road to recovery.

Were you lulled into a false sense of security?

"I so enjoyed being pregnant, I never really thought of life beyond my due date."

You may have felt that you would be pregnant forever. Your due date seemed such a massive hurdle to overcome. You couldn't imagine life beyond it. You got used to being pregnant and eating large amounts of food. You just didn't think about how your body would look afterwards. If this is you, remember that no stage in life lasts forever. Change is a part of life. Enjoy the present, but always keep an eye on the future and avoid unnecessary stress by being prepared for the inevitability of change.

Did you take into consideration your build, your birth weight, your prepregnancy weight, and whether or not this is your first baby?

"I gained forty pounds in my pregnancy. The doctor said this was fine for my build."

"I've still got ten pounds to lose from my last baby."

All these factors can determine how much you gain. If you are large and big-boned, a weight gain of twenty-five to thirty-five pounds may be a little too restrictive. You will need to gain more. Also, your baby's size may be influenced by your own birth weight. If you were born large or small, your baby might be, too. If you were overweight before you got pregnant, you may tend to put on more weight during your pregnancy. If you were underweight, you will need to put on more weight. And finally, if this is your second, third, or fourth child, remember that most women gain an average of five pounds for each baby. Unfortunately, they don't tend to lose it.

How old are you?

"I'm thirty-nine. Is it going to be harder for me to manage my weight?"

You are also more likely to gain more weight the older you are when you have a baby. As a woman ages her metabolic rate slows down. It's easier to gain weight. For more information about metabolism and weight gain, see Part Five.

Did you exercise throughout your pregnancy?

"I used to jog every day, but I was so worried about miscarrying that I stopped exercising altogether."

You may also have decreased your activity levels too much when you got pregnant. Perhaps you were still influenced by the old school of thought that recommended that pregnant women keep as quiet as possible and don't exert themselves. If you slowed down too much, you wouldn't have used so much energy, and weight gain is likely. You do need to slow down when you are pregnant, but not too much. Unless you are high-risk, activity during pregnancy is beneficial for you and for baby. It will help you manage your weight, too.

Did you just have bad luck?

"In my first pregnancy I put on forty pounds. So when I got pregnant the second time, I did everything right. I ate sensibly. I exercised. I meditated to stay calm. And I still put on forty pounds."

And finally, you might have gained too much weight for no real reason at all. It's just one of those things. Whatever you do, the weight still piles on. The only possible explanation is that your biochemistry is such that your body has as much fat stored as possible to ensure adequate milk production for baby. You won't be able to lose much of the weight you have gained until you wean. If this is the case, it is still vital for your health and your baby's health that you make wise food and exercise choices to prevent an even greater weight gain.

As long as you know that you are doing all you can to make sure both you and your baby-to-be are healthy, the only answer is to accept your body's wisdom. Your body knows what it needs to create the miracle of new life. And for some women, this is to store just a little more fat than is usual.

You are gaining weight for the best possible reason.

A healthy diet and regular exercise can help you gain the required amount of weight slowly and gradually. But all too often the excitement of having a baby, bodily changes, and morning sickness throw things off balance. You might gain twenty pounds in your first trimester, for example, or not gain anything at all. You may go crazy in the second trimester and gain far too much, and so on. If you do find that your weight gain has strayed significantly from what you planned, you can still get back on track. Remember, though, that you can't stop gaining weight. Your baby-to-be can't thrive on that. He needs a steady supply of nutrients from you daily. You should talk to your doctor and establish how much weight you still need to gain and try not to go over that amount.

Whatever stage you are in pregnancy, weight gain can be alarming. Try always to bear in mind that the changes in your body shape have a good cause: Your body is bring a new life into the world, and that's a huge amount of work. There is an explanation for every pound gained during your pregnancy. You can help your body by treating it well and giving it what it needs. Too much or too little food is not going to help it. Too much or too little exercise is not good for it, either. Nor are negative emotions and hating the way you look.

All of us will have weight to lose postpartum. For some of us it will be five pounds, for others thirty. Part Five will show you how you can shed those excess pounds after baby is born, but if you ate a healthy diet and kept your weight gain within the weight range that was right for you during your pregnancy, you'll find it much easier to lose that baby fat.

If it all seems overwhelming at present, take heart. What seems so vivid now—the morning sickness, the backache, the weight gain—will be forgotten. There may soon come a time when you find it hard to even remember being pregnant. Yes, you have gained weight, and this weight gain could be a few pounds or twenty pounds. But as you hold your baby in your arms, you might just realize what a miracle your body has performed and how everything, even the nausea, swollen ankles, and extra weight, was worth it.

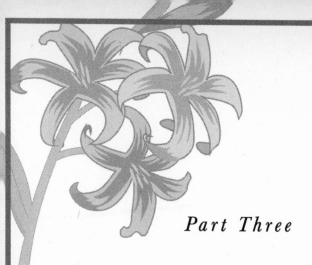

Part Three

Heavy with Child:
What Babies Do to Our Bodies

What causes the baby blues?
Still looking pregnant a month after delivery.

12

I Still Look Pregnant

CONGRATULATIONS. YOU ARE ENTERING THE "FOURTH TRIMESTER" (VICKI Iovine, *Girlfriends' Guide to the First Year of Motherhood*, Perigee, 1997). This is the trimester the books don't tell you much about. Your baby is born. You still look pregnant.

Madonna, Rachel Hunter, and Demi Moore went from maternity dresses to sexy dresses in a matter of weeks. And by so doing, they made the rest of us feel like failures. But what we seem to forget is that losing weight and getting back in shape is much easier when you have lots of money, a full-time nanny, several personal trainers, your own gym, and a personal nutritionist at your disposal. This chapter will tell you what real moms can realistically expect in terms of weight loss in the postpartum period. Here are some extracts, concerning weight loss in the postpartum period, from the journal of a friend of mine I'll call Samantha, age 34.

Week 1

Mary was born on Christmas Eve. She weighed 7 lbs 5 oz. I also gave birth to a placenta and lots of fluid. I'm 16 pounds lighter than I was a week ago. But I have to lose 18 pounds to get to my prepregnancy weight of 120. I'm 5 ft 3 in. There isn't much time to think about my weight now, though. I'm not really focused on diet at all. As for exercise, that's the last thing on my mind. I wouldn't want to even if I could. My doctor says I should wait until my six-week checkup. I've got stitches between my legs anyway, and they make walking to the restroom difficult. I don't think I'll ever be able to jog again. My fitness goal at present is to make it through the day without collapsing into tears from exhaustion.

Week 2

I'm so tired. I thought babies were supposed to nap for four to five hours. Why doesn't mine? I'm not as swollen as last week and have been able to get around a little more. The trouble with being more mobile is that it forces me to think about how I look. A brief glance in the mirror has confirmed my worst suspicions. I'm flabby all over. My stomach sags and my bottom hangs. I still look about five months pregnant. Which is better, I suppose, than the seven months pregnant I looked last week. I'm still wearing my maternity leggings and baggy jumpers. Have grown attached to them somehow and don't seem able to wear anything else. Mary was two weeks early, so I never had time to say goodbye to being pregnant. I miss having her inside me. I am not sure if I am going to be a good mom. Nothing seems to be coming naturally.

All-time low. I stood in front of the mirror for the first time. I look pregnant. May never go out of the house again.

Week 3

I can't seem to stop sweating and I'm constantly in the restroom. Things are looking up. I have lost 5 pounds. I don't look quite so pregnant. My bust looks exciting, too. I've gone from a B to a C cup. I think I'm going to like having a cleavage. The only problem is it gets uncomfortable when I'm active. Need to buy a whole new set of supportive bras. Have been told that breastfeeding helps you lose weight. I'm going to breastfeed for years.

Week 4

What's happened? I've gained 3 pounds again. I felt terrific when I got up. Really skinny. I nursed and then weighed myself. Am going to buy a set of electronic scales. Am convinced mine have something wrong with them or that the needle gets stuck. . . .

Feel terrible. The electronic scales say I am even heavier. Two pounds heavier than my old scales. I feel such a failure. According to these scales I'm 137 lbs. I suppose I'm not doing that badly, considering I gained 34 pounds, but I still feel quite depressed about my weight.

Week 5

I went for a little jog today. I know my doctor said wait till I see her next week, but I felt I could cope. I ran for twenty minutes. I don't think I went very far, just around the block, but it didn't matter. It felt great to move again. I took Mary in her stroller—it was delightful to watch her sleep. In the evening, though, I started bleeding again. Knew I shouldn't have pushed myself. My body just isn't ready yet.

Weight Loss in the First Six Weeks

According to Eileen Behan in *Eat Well, Lose Weight While Breast-feeding* (Villard Books, 1992, p. 65), "There are no hard and fast rules about weight loss after birth, but one hour after delivery the average mother can expect to lose about thirteen and a half pounds."

You should expect immediate weight loss in the first week. It just won't be the twenty or so pounds you had hoped for. Weight loss after delivery will break down as follows, if you gained the recommended twenty-five to thirty-five pounds: your baby, five to ten pounds, and the placenta, one to two pounds. Remember, though—postpartum weight loss is unpredictable. You may find that you deliver a nine-pound baby and only have a weight loss of twelve or so pounds. You may find that you deliver a six-pound baby and have an immediate weight loss of fifteen pounds.

Generally, though, by the end of the second week postpartum you should have lost another five to ten pounds of body fluid. Since baby is no longer relying on your blood supply, your own blood volume and fluid levels return to normal. A major part of the weight loss now is water weight. Increased perspiration and urination begins about twelve hours after delivery and continues right up to about eight weeks post-partum. Expect to sweat a lot in the first few weeks. Some women may find that the sweating goes on much longer—several months longer. As you're sweating so much, you'll probably feel very thirsty. Your body wants to make up for the fluid loss.

You may wake up drenched in sweat. This sweating is a healthy sign of postpartum hormonal readjustment, especially a drop in your estrogen levels. This could cause night sweats and hot flashes. Hot flashes may also occur when you start to breastfeed. A slight fever is possible, too. An elevation in temperature is common during the first twenty-four hours after delivery. But if your temperature rises higher than 100.4°F for any two days during the first ten days postpartum, consult your doctor.

Not all women will lose body fluid in the early weeks, though. "I couldn't believe it," says Jennifer, age 32, a week after delivery. "I expected to lose more than just 10 pounds." Sometimes fluid retention occurs and you won't see a weight loss. This can be frustrating. Give your body time and it should adjust. If it doesn't, consult your doctor.

In the early weeks you may feel as if you are still pregnant. However much weight you have lost, you'll probably find that you still want to wear your maternity clothes. I got passionately attached to my red maternity dress and found it impossible to put on anything else. Don't go clothes shopping now. It's depressing! Your waist may be nonexistent and your belly flabby. Your uterus will take about six weeks to go back to its original size, but your abdominals could be slack for even longer and take quite a while to get some tone back.

Don't be disappointed with yourself if you have not lost as much weight as you hoped. You have not done anything wrong. Now is not the time to get serious about weight loss, especially if you are breast-feeding. Give yourself a break. You have enough on your plate at the moment with a new baby to care for. Your body has just done something amazing. Don't start to criticize yourself for not being skinny. Ignore all the magazine covers with skinny models holding tiny four-week-old babies, or celebrities in skin-tight designer dresses two weeks after giving birth to twins. Their lives are not your life.

At the moment bonding with your child and building your life as a family is what matters. Take a vacation from the diet mentality of restrictions and prohibitions. Eat good food to nourish you and your baby. You need the nutrients to recover from childbirth. Start a gentle walking schedule to make you feel stronger. See what your weight settles at around six weeks and take things from there.

Your Weight at Six Weeks to Six Months

"Six weeks after my delivery, frustrated, tired, and hormonally challenged, I sobbed and sobbed because I still could not put on a pair of size 14 pants. My middle just bulged out of them. Wasn't I supposed to be in shape by now?" Karen, age 37

When you leave the hospital with your brand new baby, your doctor asked you to schedule a six-week postpartum checkup. The weeks have flown by, and now you've reached that magic date circled in your diary. It's six weeks postpartum. Isn't that when you are supposed to have got your figure back? Why have you still got so much weight to lose?

Very few women return to their prepregnancy weight postpartum. In fact, you are unlikely to feel "normal" again for many months to come. "Whether you're three or thirteen pounds overweight during the first six months, you may be dismayed at your postpartum figure," writes Paula Siegal in *The Next Nine Months: A Guide to Your Body After Giving Birth* (Penguin, 1996, p. 155) Some of us can lose all the weight quickly, but the majority of us will experience weight struggles perhaps similar to those Samantha writes about her in diary.

Week 6

I still have 17 pounds to lose. It's depressing. I don't like the way I look. Everybody says how lovely my little girl is. Then they look at me with a kind of pity in their eyes. I must look dreadful. I feel dreadful.

My doctor says I am fine. I can go back to my normal activities. I can have sex again. I can exercise. She said I should start slowly, though, and build up. Strange, but now I have been given the go-ahead, I feel like exercising even less. As for sex, I'm too tired. What I wouldn't give to sleep more than four hours.

Week 7

I've been trying to get my abdominals back in shape this week. The first time I could only manage twenty crunches, but by the end of the week I was doing fifty. If I am ever going to wear any of my old clothes again, I have to get my abs into some kind of shape. Perhaps I should sign up for an exercise class? I'd have to get a sitter, though, and I don't think I'm ready for that yet. I'd just worry about my baby. I do need to get some kind of motivation going, though. My postpartum shape-up is just not happening. Still 15 pounds to lose.

I saw a magazine article on "sexy moms." Pamela Anderson Lee is sexy. In fact, she said she felt sexier than ever and being a mom is no excuse to let yourself go. I hate her. I think I have every right to look frumpy. With burping, diaper changes, and constant nursing how can I look my best?

Week 8

My back aches. Those car seats are so heavy. When I carry mine it scrapes me in the shins. Am not weighing myself this week. I feel fat. My jogging is getting better, though. Made half an hour yesterday and no bleeding. Have really started to bond with Mary. Can't imagine life without her now.

Week 9

I'm getting there slowly. Twelve pounds till I reach my target weight. Can even fit into some of my old clothes again. The ones without a waistline. Am trying to jog for half an hour and do fifty crunches a day. I am determined not to buy a new set of clothes. If I do I think I'll just give up on the weight loss thing altogether.

The trouble is my appetite is huge. I mean really huge. I want to eat all the time. I'm sure that's why I'm not losing the weight.

Week 10

My scales are stuck. I haven't lost any weight again this week. Think I am so hungry because of the breastfeeding. Have a short vacation next week at my in-laws. Think it will be good for me. There won't be any scales to tell me I'm not losing weight.

Week 11

Great to be away. I was nervous at first, but Mary didn't fuss too much. I also got some time for me. I went for long runs (about 45 mins) and went to a gym. By the end of the week I was ready to leave, though. I missed time alone with Mary

Week 12

Can't face the scales. I should try to walk more. I should take her for long walks. Time is always the problem, though. There is always so much to do. Mountains of laundry. Bottles to boil. Beds to be made. Letters and calls to make. I have to decide about work soon. I have no idea what I am going to do. I am so much in mother mode that I can't think of doing anything else right now.

Week 20

My weight is around 130 pounds or so. That means I've still got ten pounds to go. Perhaps I have got more muscle now with all the lifting I have to do? Perhaps, though, I need to cut back on the cookies and candy bars midafternoon?

Ten pounds to go isn't that bad is it? Perhaps getting back to 120 is unrealistic? Perhaps I should aim for 125.

Week 25

I have no idea how much I weigh. Think I have lost a few pounds, though, as my trousers fit better. I do worry about my weight, but more and more lately I just forget to stand on the scales. Mary's beautiful smile makes me forget.

At six weeks any weight that is left above your prepregnancy level is fat and breast tissue. If you gained twenty-five to thirty-five pounds, you will be around five to eighteen pounds heavier than you were before baby. You may not look pregnant anymore, but you will probably feel flabby. You might have problems trying to fit into your prepregnancy wardrobe. You can't zip your jeans. Skirts seem unbearably tight. Your shirts feel strained.

From six weeks, the dramatic weight loss after pregnancy is over. For the next few months, most women find it hard to shift any weight at all. Understanding why this happens may help. Your body is still in baby mode. It will cling to that extra fat you have gained for the baby's sake. Your body is preserving fat stores for milk production in case of famine or disaster. You can expect to stay in this baby mode until you start your normal menstrual cycle again. A lot depends on the return of the menstrual cycle. If you are bottle feeding, you can expect menses to return at around six to eight weeks. If you are breastfeeding, periods may not start until you have weaned, so onset of menstruation for nursing mothers is hard to predict. Some moms find that when their feedings are less frequent in the later months of breastfeeding, they get their menses back. This usually doesn't happen for a few months post-partum, but pregnancy during nursing in the first few months could happen. Nursing is no guarantee of contraception.

The return of the menstrual cycle is significant for weight loss postpartum because it signals the final return of your body to its prepregnancy hormonal state, and weight loss should be easier. Many moms I spoke to said that after months of weight maintenance, they suddenly lost a few pounds when their cycles returned. Some also lost weight when they weaned because milk-producing breasts can add several pounds to the scale.

Six weeks is not the date you should set yourself for being fully recovered both physically and emotionally. Six weeks, though, is a turning point. Around this time you may gradually start to feel human again. You may still feel overweight, tired, and sore from childbirth, but feeling normal again won't seem such a remote possibility. As for the extra breast and fat tissue you are left with after six weeks, how long you take to lose that depends on your lifestyle, how much you gained when you were pregnant, whether you are breastfeeding, and whether your cycles have returned. If you think in terms of nine months on, nine months off, you would be about right. But remember how different we all are. How different our lives are. How we lose or gain weight at different rates. Some can lose it in the first six weeks. Some lose it in the first three months. Others take six months to a year. Some never lose it at all.

Few return to exactly the same weight they were before baby. Some end up below their prepregnancy weight, but most of us end up about five pounds heavier. Most women notice that their bodies have changed in some way. Some think it changes for the better. Others think it changes for the worse. Here's what some moms told me about their weight loss after six weeks:

"I gained 42 pounds with this baby. So far I've lost about 38 pounds. Those last 4 or 5 pounds are going to be hard. I think my body had changed for the worse. Everything's in different proportions. I do exercise three times a week for about an hour. My diet is healthy because I'm breastfeeding." Linda, age 33, at week 10 postpartum

"I'm about 5 ft 2 in and I gained nearly 45 pounds with this baby. In the first week I lost about 10 pounds and then another 10 in the next few weeks. I couldn't exercise at all for the first eight weeks due to a cesarean. I've lost a total of 25 pounds now. I don't like my post-baby body at all. I exercise three to four times a week. I do 30 minutes of cardio and weight training and hour-long walks. My trainer says I have to persist but I get despondent. My husband encourages me to exercise. I can't diet because I'm breastfeeding." Margaret, age 35, at week 12 postpartum

"I'm 5 ft 7 in and before I got pregnant I was around 145 pounds. I gained 28 pounds. Twenty pounds came off in the first six weeks but after that nothing. I'm a little unhappy about it. The extra weight makes me feel older. I've got a fuller bust and seem firmer in the hips. Baby doesn't make it impossible for me to exercise, but he makes it easier to find an excuse. I've never enjoyed exercise much. I could diet 'cause I'm not breastfeeding, but so far have not found the motivation." Lucy, age 27, at week 16 postpartum

"I only gained 20 pounds with my pregnancy. I'm 5 ft 4 in and was 130 pounds before I had the baby. In the first six weeks I lost about ten pounds. Then the pounds slipped away. I'm now down to 125 pounds. I'm not breastfeeding anymore. My milk supply stopped at around four weeks. This is my second baby. I work full-time. I guess I'm losing weight fast 'cause I don't get time to eat. I'm constantly tired. Have not started my exercise routine yet so feel quite unfit. I don't much like the look of my body. Everything seems a bit flabby." Louise, age 28, at week 20 postpartum

Weight Loss Six Months Postpartum

"There's long been a popular belief among new mothers," writes Jacqueline Shannon in *The New Mother's Body Book* (Contemporary Books, 1994, p. 38) "that fat gained during pregnancy is somehow different from other body fat and is therefore difficult to shed."

There might be a grain of truth in this, but only until your menstrual cycle starts again. After that, fat is fat, whether you gained it in pregnancy or not. Perhaps the reason why so many of us think pregnancy fat is somehow different is because with a baby to care for there seems to be so little time now to do anything about it. What's more, extra fat in women tends to go straight to our hips and thighs and rear, whether we are pregnant or not pregnant. Researchers are coming to the conclusion that fat gained here is more difficult to get rid of than in any other part of the body because it is harder to break down for use as energy—except, perhaps, if you are breastfeeding, when the body does turn to fat below the waist. (There is a school of thought that believes breastfeeding offers a great opportunity to rid yourself of fat on your thighs—an opportunity that you may not get again.)

Fat cells in the lower body are unfortunately designed for long-term holding. That's why it's so hard to lose weight there. There is some good news about the pear-shaped figure, though. Weight gained below the waist is associated with a lower risk of heart disease, diabetes, high blood pressure, and even breast cancer. It is weight gained in the waist that seems to raise the risk of heart disease, because waistline fat is metabolically active and is likely to end up circulating in your bloodstream as fatty acid.

Don't be surprised if at several months or years postpartum you are still carrying extra weight below the belt. One survey showed that as long as eighteen months after delivery, up to 40 percent of women were still an average of nine pounds heavier than their prepregnancy weight. Studies have also shown that if weight is not lost in the first year postpartum it is likely to become permanent.

But would you have stayed the same weight even if you hadn't gotten pregnant? As we age, we tend to gradually put on weight anyway—about two or three pounds every ten years. This is due not only to lowering activity levels as we age, but to the work of female hormones that prepare us for pregnancy and menopause. Think about how long it is since you had your baby—perhaps one year or two. The chances are that you might have gained a few extra pounds anyway.

Now you have seen what you can expect in terms of weight loss postpartum, let's now examine what you can expect your body to look like.

13

Your Postbaby Body

WEIGHT LOSS IS NOT THE ONLY BODILY CHANGE POSTPARTUM. THERE ARE other changes to adjust to and discomforts to deal with, all of which affect your appearance, your mood, your body image, and your self-esteem. Let's take a look at your postpartum body in the early weeks, months, and years that follow. (See Figure 8)

The Early Weeks

YOUR STOMACH

Immediately after delivery, you will still look very pregnant. Your stomach will not be flat. You won't notice it when you are lying down, but you will when you get up. The uterus, which has expanded to protect your baby these nine months, will return to a normal size quickly. It will shrink from about two pounds to two ounces. Not as quickly as straight after delivery, though.

After two weeks, your uterus will have contracted to the point that it can't be felt in the abdomen, but it will take about six weeks to fully contract. The contractions of your uterus as it shrinks are called afterpains. They are similar to menstrual cramps and last a few days. If you are breastfeeding the hormone oxytocin speeds up the process. You'll probably feel afterpains at the start of each nursing session. They should disappear after the first few days. A heating pad on the abdomen might help if they really bother you.

An enlarged uterus is not the only reason your stomach bulges and you may have no waist. Pregnancy and childbirth have weakened

FIGURE 8: YOUR POST-BABY BODY—COMMON COMPLAINTS (WKS. 1-6)

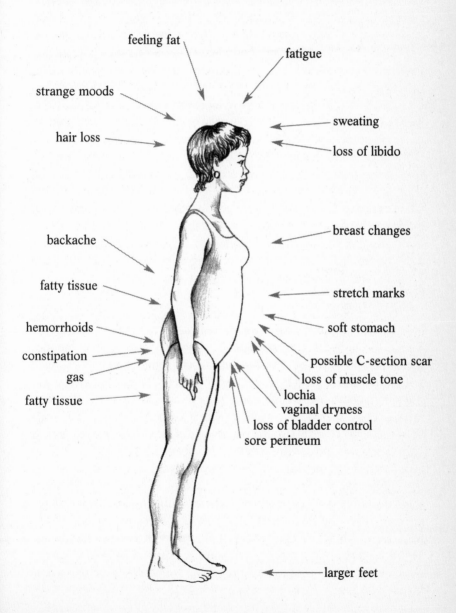

feeling fat

fatigue

strange moods

sweating

hair loss

loss of libido

backache

breast changes

fatty tissue

stretch marks

hemorrhoids

soft stomach

constipation

possible C-section scar

gas

loss of muscle tone

fatty tissue

lochia

vaginal dryness

loss of bladder control

sore perineum

larger feet

your abdominal muscles. That's why elimination can be hard right now—your stomach muscles are too weak to assist you. It's also why you have to sit using your hands—your stomach muscles can't support you yet. For a while these muscles will continue to hang loose until diet, exercise, a good posture, and time help them return to a firmer shape.

During pregnancy your abdominal muscles can stretch so greatly that the two connected sheaths of muscles running from breastbone to pelvis (the recti muscles) often separate. (See Figure 9.) This is called diastasis. Diastasis occurs a little in all pregnant women, but for some there can be a major tear. A tear usually occurs in women who gain an excessive amount of weight during pregnancy. If you can place three or more fingers into this tear during or after pregnancy, chances are you are going to have significant problems postpartum. Pain in the abdomen and back is likely, too. Strengthening the abdominals is vital so that the gap closes. For a while you may need to wear an abdominal binder prescribed by a doctor or physical therapist. To find out if you have diastasis, lie on your back with your knees bent. Put your fingers 1 to 2 inches below your belly button, fingers pointing to feet. Lift your head and feel in the tissue in the center of your abdomen.

CONSTIPATION

If you feel out of shape, heavy constipation can make you feel even worse. In the first few weeks bowels will be sluggish as your muscles regain their former tone. Constipation is very common in the first three weeks. It's hard to push because of your slack abdominal muscles, especially if you have had a C section. Progesterone, which is still lingering in your body after delivery, also makes it harder to return to normal bowel activity. There is also the psychological factor. You may approach your first bowel movement with fear. Hemorrhoids aside, you could be concerned about rupturing stitches from an episiotomy or C section.

Either before or after baby, 70 percent of women get hemorrhoids: painful, itchy swollen veins that are either outside or inside the anus. To ease the discomfort of hemorrhoids, warm sitz baths may help. Hemorrhoid ointments such as Preparation H can ease things. Try to eat fiber and drink lots of water. Constipation makes hemorrhoids worse. If this doesn't help, try stool softeners or doctor-recommended laxatives. Try not to strain with your bowel movements. Give yourself plenty of time. Make sure you thoroughly cleanse the area after

FIGURE 9: DIASTASIS

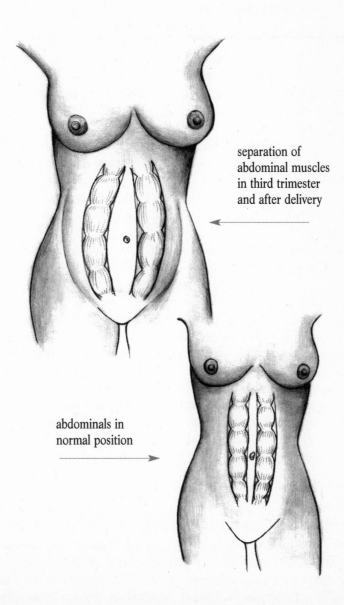

separation of
abdominal muscles
in third trimester
and after delivery

abdominals in
normal position

a bowel movement. If sitting is agony, use a hemorrhoid cushion. The good news is that hemorrhoids do tend to disappear in a few weeks after delivery. The bad news is that once you have had them, you are more likely to get them again.

FREQUENT URINATION

Your bladder has been treated a bit roughly during pregnancy and delivery. First it was squeezed, and then it was pushed aside. You may experience a variety of problems with urination in these early days. The problems are temporary, though, and normal bladder control will return. You might find that you can't urinate, or that you are urinating constantly, or that you leak when you cough or laugh. If you are not aware of your bloated bladder in the first few days because of anes-thetic, a catheter may be inserted. This is a simple procedure in which a thin tube (catheter) is guided up the bladder so that urine can flow out into an attached receptacle. This will be used also if you want to urinate but can't.

Sensation in the bladder usually returns a few days after delivery. And when it does, you will know it. Now you'll be wanting to urinate frequently as your body tries to rid itself of excess fluid. At times you'll feel like you are living in the bathroom. Many women say that their bladders are never as strong again after pregnancy. Some of us may experience stress incontinence, which is the inability to hold urine. You might find yourself wearing sanitary pads for urine flow not menstrual flow. Exercise and muscle toning help remedy the problem. (See Chapter Twenty-three for more information.) It's important that you go when the urge hits you—don't hold it. When you do go, make sure you fully empty your bladder. Certain foods and drinks, such as coffee, can make the problem worse. If leakage is excessive, consult your doctor. The very last resort is drugs and surgery.

ACHES AND PAINS

After delivery you'll feel bruised and sore all over, especially in your perineum. This is the area between your vagina and rectum. If you had an episiotomy, you may feel quite uncomfortable. There could be pain, swelling, and itching. To ease the discomfort of swelling, use the ice pack your doctor gives you. Wear it for the first twenty-four hours. Then take warm or cold sitz baths. Use the anesthetic spray your doctor gives you, too. Keep your perineum clean. Change sanitary pads often, and every time you go to the bathroom squirt clean with a bottle spray or water. Stitches will be absorbed by the body in ten days to four weeks. By the second or third week, you won't feel so much pain, just soreness. In time the soreness will fade, too.

Backache is likely, too, in these early days and weeks. Remember how pregnancy changed your center of gravity. You swayed back when you walked. Now your back has to adjust again. Your abdominal muscles won't be giving it much help right now. You'll have to start lifting your baby around soon, and this strains the back even more. Don't be surprised if backache strikes. To help ease the pain, sit with your feet up whenever you can. Try to get your knees higher than your waist when you sit. Shift your weight from foot to foot when you stand. Observe proper body mechanics when you bend or lift things or get up. Most important of all, watch your posture. Stretching and strengthening exercises for your back could help, too. Getting out of bed can be very painful if your back and perineum are sore. A few adjustments will help you ease the discomfort. Use your arms for leverage, not your lower body. Use the muscles of the pelvic floor as a splint for your perineum when you sit, and sit on a cushion or a rubber ring to ease the pain.

Headaches are common if you had an epidural anesthetic. Doctors don't know why this happens. Staying flat on your back seems to ease the pain. Consult your doctor if the pain continues for more than a few days.

FATIGUE

You may feel exhausted after delivery—too tired even to hold your baby. Or you could feel very alert and excited: you can't sleep and rest; you want company. Never mind the fact that you have probably been awake for two days—you want to see your baby. You want to talk about your delivery. You are eager to nurse. To get started. This energy spurt may even last a few days. I was up walking and shopping on the second day after my baby was born. On the fourth day I disintegrated into a heap of tears and fears. I was exhausted. The tremendous body changes I had experienced caught up with me. "Expect fatigue to set in, whether it's three minutes or three days after childbirth." (Jacqueline Shannon, *The New Mother's Body Book*, Contemporary Books, 1994, p. 15)

The best way to cope with fatigue is to make sure you are eating a healthy diet and getting all your nutrients. Lack of iron can make many of us feel fatigued. Also be patient. All new parents are chronically sleep-deprived in the first weeks. Be kind to yourself. Nap when baby naps, whatever time of day it is. Accept help from others whenever you can.

BLEEDING

We all laughed at the gigantic sanitary pads and hospital underwear the instructor showed us at the prenatal class. I didn't laugh about them after delivery. They became essential underwear!

Lochia is the term used to refer to the bloody discharge you will have in the first weeks postpartum. It consists of blood from where the placenta was attached and the lining of the uterus. The blood starts bright red, but then it can turn brown or even clear. Most of the lochia is expelled in the first few days, but expect to bleed for about three to six weeks. If you start to get too active too soon, expect your flow to get heavier. Use this as a warning sign to slow down.

If your discharge has a foul odor and causes itching and irritation, you could have an infection. Consult your doctor. Don't use tampons to absorb the discharge. Inserting anything into the vagina can increase your chance of introducing bacteria, which could lead to infection.

YOUR TEETH AND EYES

High levels of progesterone during pregnancy can alter blood vessels in your mouth. Gum disease is more likely both during and after pregnancy. This can probably be prevented if proper oral hygiene is observed. Hormonal changes can affect your eyes, too. You may have had problems with contact lenses when you were pregnant. Your eyes are not permanently altered by pregnancy. They will settle down in about six months.

VARICOSE VEINS

You could get varicose veins in the legs. Like hemorrhoids, they do improve in a few weeks, but you need to be careful from now on. If you got spider veins on your arms and legs during pregnancy, they should fade in a week or so postpartum.

C-SECTION RECOVERY

Every cesarean is different, but here is a brief guide to your body for the first few days and months. C-section recovery is a bit slower than a normal vaginal delivery, but rates of recovery differ. I talked to some women who had pain for the first few days in their abdomens. I talked to others who needed pain prescriptions for a few weeks. I talked to others who had minimal discomfort and were back to their normal routines in two weeks.

There are special considerations if you deliver by cesarean, but most of the aspects of postpartum recovery outlined here are the same. The first day is the most difficult. You may need pain relief. If you want to breast-feed, you may need to pump until you are off medication. Bear in mind that when you do start nursing, you will feel the uterine contractions more sharply. You won't be able to eat the first day or two and will be offered liquids only. Your catheter is usually removed the first day and you will be encouraged to go to the bathroom. Bladder sensitivity and normal bowel function may take a while to function normally again. Gas may cause you pain. Try to walk when you can and avoid carbonated drinks. Only when you can pass gas naturally will you be able to go on a regular diet again. You can expect to spend the three to four nights of your hospital stay learning how to sit and stand and walk.

It might be quite painful for you to find a nursing style that is comfortable while the incision heals. You'll need help in the early days positioning your baby correctly and burping your baby. You will get a bloody discharge, but it might be lighter than a vaginal delivery discharge. Despite the trauma of surgery, your body will not generally suffer the same stresses to the vagina or pelvic floor. Your uterus and abdominals, however, will obviously take longer to heal. They were not only stretched, but cut as well. Cesarean sections heal fast, but you need to be especially careful to take it easy at least for the first six weeks. Still, easing back into activity is an important part of recovery. Don't expect to stay in bed for weeks on end.

Gradually the incision will feel less tender and ache less when you are sitting and standing. However, expect to feel twinges when you use your abdominals for months afterwards. The incision might get itchy. As the weeks pass, even though your incision isn't as sore as it used to be, your stomach just won't feel the same. This is because it takes a long time for cut nerve endings to heal. Your abdomen should feel normal when they finally heal.

Although it takes a few weeks for the scar to heal properly, when it does, the uterus and abdominals are as strong as those of a woman who has delivered vaginally. If you want to try for a vaginal delivery for your next baby this will be possible. C sections are becoming so routine now that the risk of complication is very, very low, although occasionally they can occur. As for the scar, it might stay with you, but many women say they have trouble locating it a year after surgery.

By far the most frustrating thing in the early days will be the lack of mobility. You won't be able to get around for the first few days. You have to lie down to hold your baby. You are still weak and sore. You might feel that you won't be able to cope with the baby once you leave the hospital. Ask for help if you are really worried. Remember, you are recovering from a major surgery. Give yourself time to heal.

Whether you had a vaginal delivery or a cesarean, there will probably be times when you will wonder if it really was worth putting your body through all this. You may feel that recovery takes far longer than you hoped it would. As your six-week checkup draws near, you probably won't feel anywhere near fully recovered. You are not alone. Few, if any women, feel great at six weeks. Whenever you feel overwhelmed, take a long look at your baby. It certainly was worth it. And if you are still in those early weeks of sleepless nights, sore nipples, and crying, just wait a few weeks until your baby starts smiling at you. That smile will light up your world.

Six Weeks to Six Months

If you read any book or magazine that tells you that you should be back in shape by six weeks after delivery, burn it. You don't need this pressure. It takes most of us far longer. Six weeks is how long it takes for your reproductive organs to return to their prepregnancy state. "But evidence is mounting that it takes a great many women a good deal longer than that before they feel like their normal selves." (Jacqueline Shannon, *New Mother's Body Book*, Contemporary Books, 1994, p. 17)

Few of us will feel totally recovered physically at six weeks. As well as weight loss, other factors need to be taken into account. Muscle tone, weight redistribution, and skin elasticity play key roles in how quickly you can recover and get in shape.

MUSCLE TONE

Muscles are stretched when you are pregnant, especially in the abdominal and pelvic floor areas. If you want to have a sleek figure, you need to work on regaining your muscle tone. Muscles need to be strong and toned to support your body structure. If they are weak, you will look out of shape. To get your figure back, you need to get active and start strengthening them again. (See Chapter 23 for more information.)

WEIGHT REDISTRIBUTION

Progesterone during pregnancy encourages fat storage in the lower part of your body. This is to make sure you have enough nutrients to feed your baby when he or she is born. Progesterone levels fall off after birth, but you will still have this excess weight, which can take a few months to lose. You'll see most of this new weight gain on the lower part of your body from the waist down. Pregnancy can also change the curvature of your spine, and this may not correct itself after birth. How you walk, stand, sit—how you carry yourself—may now be slightly different. You could even be a little shorter. Good posture has never been so important.

YOUR SKIN

When you are pregnant, your skin stretches. The older you are, the longer it will take for skin tone to return. Skin becomes less elastic as we age. It could take some time for skin to shrink back, so be patient if you see loose skin on your stomach, hips, and breasts. In some cases, though, skin is never as firm as it was before.

Most of the lack of tone in your belly is due to stretched skin and muscle. A few weeks after delivery, skin will settle into a slack resting position and you will have a soft potbelly. You can get your waistline back, but it will take time and effort. I was a fitness instructor and I told women in prenatal classes that it would take them about two months to get their waists back. After having my own baby I was a little less optimistic. It took me about six months. Some experts believe that after childbirth the abdominal muscles are slacker. They will never be as flat. Other experts disagree. They say you can get them back in shape. The firmer they were before childbirth, the easier this is.

Yet another reason to avoid putting on too much weight when you are pregnant is that if you stretch your skin to its limit, you will get stretch marks, probably on your stomach and breasts. These will initially be red, but they will fade to a silvery-white mark. Stretch marks surprisingly seem to occur more often in younger women, perhaps because older skin is not so tight to begin with. If you have grown soft little pads of skin tissue under the arms, or on your breasts or neck, they won't go away after delivery.

Permanent Postpartum Bodily Changes

Here's what some moms of toddlers said about their bodies postpartum:

> "I feel attractive, but not in the same way I used to. It's very hard to describe. My appearance is definitely not as important to me as it used to be. I love being a mom more than I love being slim."

> "I'm still about 7 pounds over my target weight. I have no muscle tone in my stomach anymore and my feet are bigger."

> "People always say they can't believe I had a baby. My body didn't change that much, but my hair did. It got really curly. Another change I noticed was that I get sick a lot more than I did before."

> "I love my postbaby body. I'm stronger and slimmer than I have ever been. I'm actually lower in weight than before I had my kids."

> "My body has changed for the worse. Everything is in a different place. I've lost my waistline. I've gone up a clothes size. My breasts have shrunk. I think I look much older."

"Before I got pregnant it was easier for me to lose weight and stay in shape. I just never have the time now, and besides, doesn't having a baby make your hips expand?"

"I have far more body confidence now than I ever had. My body did something really wonderful."

Contrary to popular belief, your hips do not permanently expand after baby. Bones and muscles do not increase in size. What still may be with you is the extra layer of fat you gained during pregnancy, and your breasts may have changed shape. You may have lost muscle tone, especially in the stomach, thighs, and in the pelvic floor area. You could be a few pounds heavier and slightly fuller in figure. But this is not the end of the world. If your body has reached a weight it feels comfortable at and you are eating sensibly and exercising regularly, perhaps it is time to accept your body's wisdom and think about going up a clothes size. "There's no rule that says you must fit into your prepregnancy clothes to be attractive again." (Paula Siegal, *The Next Nine Months*, Penguin, 1996, p. 220)

Other changes you might notice are in your feet and your hair. Many women report that they get bigger feet with each pregnancy. This may have something to do with the fact that as we get older, our foot size tends to increase anyway. But the added weight of pregnancy and the role of the hormone relaxin could also be contributory factors. Your hair, which was glorious during pregnancy, may not be so glorious now. You could start shedding hair. Some women say their hair changed completely. It went curly instead of straight, or straight instead of curly. It went a couple of shades darker or a couple of shades lighter. This again has to do with hormones and hair growth patterns. Hair loss is not permanent. By the first year postpartum it should be back to normal. As for radical changes in how your hair looks, there is no evidence to support that this happens, but it is possible.

The position of the uterus will be different in a woman who has had a baby. It will be much lower. As the uterus grows during pregnancy, it stretches tissues and ligaments that support it. If you have a vaginal delivery, these stretch even more. Although the body does repair, some stretching is permanent. How much lower the uterus will be depends on how much stretching occurred, the size of the baby, and the length of your delivery. Your cervix (the opening of your uterus) will be larger, too. You may notice that vaginal discharge is heavier because of this. Your vagina will probably be a little larger, but this won't affect sexual pleasure. It usually takes about two to three months for it to have its prepregnancy muscle tone back. If you were very body aware before pregnancy, you could notice that your labia are softer and fleshier than they were before baby. They will also be maroon-colored now and not pink.

Many women say that after they have a baby, they get sicker more often. There is no evidence to support this, and it may well have to do with the fact that children with little immunity bring bugs home. Other common ailments such as headaches, aches and pains, fatigue, and digestive problems also seem to get worse. Again, this may be due to the stress of family life. Osteoporosis seems to have a higher incidence among mothers than among women who don't have babies.

It's not all bad news, though. Pregnancy can relieve menstrual problems such as PMS. It is very beneficial for women with endometriosis. It also appears to decrease the risk of breast, ovarian, uterine, endometrial, bladder, colon, and brain cancer. And pregnancy seems to make us more resilient. We can cope with pain and discomfort better. For many years before having my baby, I wanted to have my vision corrected by surgery. I was too scared. After baby I found the courage. If you've been through childbirth, you do seem more tolerant of minor aches, pains, and stresses. You definitely feel braver, as if you can cope with anything.

Even if you do manage to reach your prepregnancy weight, you won't feel the same way about your body. This is because however many months or years post partum you are, however much you exercise and diet, your body and your life have changed. You cannot get your old body back. You have a new body. One that has been through childbirth and brought a baby into your life. And if you treat this body with respect, it can be an even better body.

14

What Happened to My Breasts?

AFTER YOU HAVE HAD A BABY, YOUR BREASTS WON'T LOOK QUITE THE same. Although we seem to be the most concerned about weight gain in the lower part of the body, it's amazing how different you can feel about yourself when your breasts change shape.

> "I don't think I look good if my breasts don't look good."

> "When I lost weight, my breasts got smaller and I felt so much better about myself."

> "After I had my baby, my breasts got larger. I feel much more feminine."

During pregnancy and postpartum, your breasts will undergo a remarkable series of transformations. From the moment of conception your mammary glands start their work. In no time at all they start to grow, change shape, and develop an incredible maze of milk-producing glands. (See Figure 10) By the end of your third trimester and during nursing, your breasts will add several pounds to your scale.

To help you come to terms with your changing breasts, it is helpful to understand what actually happens to your breasts during pregnancy and postpartum.

During Pregnancy

> "I didn't enjoy gaining weight at all, but I loved what was happening to my breasts. It was wonderful to have such a full bust. It made me feel very sexy and feminine."

FIGURE 10: YOUR INCREDIBLE BREASTS (MILK PRODUCTION)

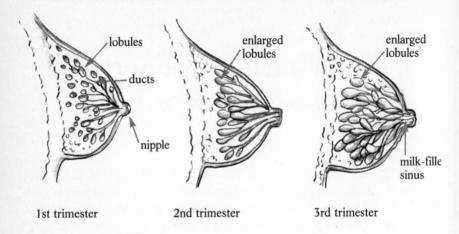

| 1st trimester | 2nd trimester | 3rd trimester |

At conception your breasts won't look that much different, but inside a lot is going on. The milk-producing network is forming. Lobes and lobules consisting of alveoli, milk-producing tissue, and milk ducts to carry milk are forming. As your pregnancy progresses, these will grow in size and quantity until the end of your pregnancy when pre-milk, called colostrum, is ready for when the baby-to-be is born. Actual milk will be produced within days of birth.

Your breasts might feel a little sore and tender in the early weeks of pregnancy as if you were about to have a menstrual period. In the first few months, you may notice that breasts seem heavier and more sensitive and that veins become more prominent. This is because of an increased blood flow to the breasts and a buildup of fatty tissue to protect the network of milk ducts and glands. Estrogen and progesterone levels increase and promote the growth of alveoli and milk ducts. If you look at your nipples now, you might detect that the areola, the area around your nipples, is darker and bigger. Nipples feel more sensitive. Small bumps on the areola, called Montgomery glands, may appear.

During the course of your pregnancy you will gain anything between one and four pounds of fat on your breasts. If you didn't have much of a cleavage before, you may enjoy having one now. Many women say how much fun it is to have a full bust when they are pregnant and how sexy it makes them feel. Others don't enjoy their breasts quite so much. They say it makes them feel self-conscious or uncomfortable.

In the second trimester, breasts continue to increase in size. Now is the time that the breastfeeding hormone prolactin makes its appearance to help the alveoli know when to produce milk. Cells in the alveoli don't actually start producing milk right now, but colostrum will be produced. Colostrum is what your baby feeds on first. It is a fluid that contains all the nutrients your baby needs for the first few days of life. Your areola will darken further and your nipples will grow more sensitive. You might even start leaking colostrum. Not all women do, though. Your breasts are as unique as you are and what happens never follows quite the same time schedule. A supportive bra is essential now, especially if you exercise. You might find that your heavier breasts make certain types of exercise uncomfortable and you have to modify. For example, instead of jogging you might need to switch to walking.

If the changes in your breasts have not been that noticeable, you can't miss them in the third trimester. Your breast size will have increased significantly, your nipples will be more erect, and your areola darker and bigger. If your baby was born, now you could give it breast milk if your breasts were stimulated by a pump or by your baby. The milk-production system continues to develop and grow throughout this trimester. Colostrum is more likely to leak. If you get any leakage, avoid scrubbing and soap, as they can irritate your nipples.

Now is the time to take breastfeeding classes if you intend to breastfeed. Breastfeeding is not as easy and as natural as many women think. I was surprised at how clumsy and clueless I felt when first trying to breastfeed my son. I didn't know how to hold him properly, how to help him latch on correctly, how long he should be at the breast, and so on. I really needed the advice of nurses and lactation consultants before and after delivery.

At Delivery

When your baby arrives, the hormone prolactin takes charge as levels of estrogen and progesterone, which had put milk production on hold previously, decrease. Your breasts will produce colostrum at first. It may take a few days for your milk to come in. Some women take one or two days; others have to wait four or five days. It is very rare for milk not to come in at all.

When your milk supply does come in, you will know it. Breasts will feel inflated like balloons. They could be hard and uncomfortable. If you don't want to nurse, not emptying the milk will prevent more production and compress the milk-producing structures. Milk will be absorbed by surrounding tissues. Compressing the breasts tightly helps this process. You might feel sore. Applying a cool compress or maybe even taking some pain relief will help.

If you do intend to nurse, you need to nurse as soon as you can after delivery. Colostrum is all that your baby needs right now, and the more you nurse, the more you stimulate your breasts to produce milk. With breastfeeding, supply and demand is the order of the day. The more your baby feeds, the more milk you have to feed him with.

Nursing

"Nursing my baby made me think about my breasts in a very different way."

"I felt uncomfortable about the whole idea of breastfeeding."

"Nursing made me far less inhibited about my body."

You may be surprised by how different you and your partner feel about your breasts when you start nursing. How they look seems less important now than how well they function, how well nourished they keep your baby. You realize that your breasts are functional organs designed not only to give sexual pleasure, but to feed your baby. You may find it difficult to accept the loss of control you have over your body when you are nursing. When baby cries or it is time for a feeding, your body goes into mother mode. Wherever you are and whatever you are doing, you start leaking. You have to stop what you are doing and nurse or pump to stop the flow. For me, nursing really brought home the fact that my body had an agenda. The rest of me had very little control over what was happening.

Breastfeeding could make you less self-conscious about your breasts if you were before. Constantly having to take out a breast and feed your baby might take away any inhibitions you may have had. If you decide to nurse in public, you may feel that feeding your hungry baby is all that matters. Your breasts can feed him, and what other people think is up to them. Besides, it is easy to use a shawl or a nursing blouse and nurse discreetly.

In the early months, you may feel pain as your breasts engorge. Engorgement takes place when you miss a feeding or wait too long to nurse. If baby is not at hand, you may have to express some milk manually or with a pump to relieve the discomfort. Watch out for nipple irritation and soreness. Warm, moist towels may help, as can nipple cream. Try to let your nipples be exposed to the air as much as you can to ensure they dry properly. Engorgement should fade in about three months when your breasts settle into a routine. When your milk supply is established, breasts will decrease in size and feel less heavy.

For many women, breastfeeding is an important part of the whole experience of pregnancy and childbirth. They would feel incomplete without it. Those intimate moments with a newborn are cherished forever. Other women, however, choose not to breastfeed because for some medical reason they can't or they are uncomfortable with the whole idea of breastfeeding. Having a baby at your breast may seem unnatural to you. You don't want that level of intimacy. You don't want the inconvenience of constant nursing. You don't want your life disrupted. You don't want to put your body through any more than it has been through already. But if you are having doubts, bear in mind that all experts agree that breast milk is best for your baby in the early months.

Weaning

"A week after I stopped nursing, my breasts looked dreadful. They had no shape at all."

When you stop nursing your baby frequently and start to wean, your milk supply soon decreases. If the milk is not used, your breasts stop producing milk. Existing milk is absorbed into the bloodstream. The ducts, alveoli, fat, and extra blood vessels contract. Your breasts will change shape again and you could lose a couple of pounds. Immediately after weaning, your breasts will look very flat and loose. They shouldn't look this exhausted forever, though; as time passes they will become more uplifted.

Your Postpregnancy Breasts

"Why didn't anyone tell me that my breasts would shrink after I had my baby."

"I had to buy a whole new wardrobe. My bust had changed so much."

"I like having fuller breasts. I had such a small bust before."

Whether you breastfeed or not, it may still take up to a year for skin to firm up again around deflated breasts. Your nipples will look fuller after pregnancy and nursing, but many moms notice that their breasts just are not the same. In general, breasts won't go back to their former shape and will look different. They could end up bigger if you didn't have much of a bust before, or smaller. Most often they look smaller. A reduction in breast size after pregnancy is known as postpartum breast atrophy. Postpartum breasts tend to look more tear-shaped and will be looser, as the stretched skin supporting the breastfeeding network never completely contracts to its former firmness.

For those of us anxious about our body image, it doesn't help that in today's society the ideal woman is supposed to not just be thin—she must have full, firm breasts as well. Unless you were born with unusual genes, this really is an impossible ideal. It's very hard to have extra fat just in your bust and not anywhere else in your body.

If you find that the shape of your breasts depresses you, exercise and healthy eating will help, but you also need to rethink your body image. There is no such thing as the perfect breast, just as there is no such thing as the perfect body. There are just different kinds of breasts and different kinds of bodies. Your breasts may have changed shape, but that doesn't mean that they or you are unattractive. They are just as attractive as they were before, but in a different way. What's more, there are benefits for breasts postpartum. You have a lower risk of breast cancer. If you nursed, you gave your child the best start in life that you could. And you have a gorgeous baby in your life. Now isn't that worth a change in cup size?

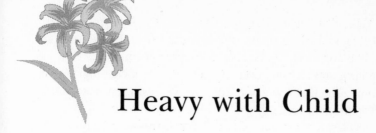

Heavy with Child

AT THE FIRST MOTHERS' GROUP I ATTENDED SHORTLY AFTER MY BABY WAS born, the instructor asked each one of us to say something about ourselves and how we felt. In a group of twelve, ten of us said we felt uncomfortable with our bodies. We didn't feel good about how we looked. We wanted to lose weight. There were comments like:

"I feel like I've lost control of my body. I feel huge."

"I just can't stand the way I look since I had my baby. I feel so flabby and out of shape."

"I'm really not happy about how out of shape I am. I have to wear baggy clothes."

"If I could just lose this weight, I know I'd feel happier about myself."

As I drove home, the sadness and regret in those women's voices stayed with me. We were all new moms. Weren't we supposed to be a little more happy? Was it really just our weight that was making us unhappy?

The Baby Blues

There is a plausible explanation for the emotional twilight zone that occurs for most of us postpartum. Most new moms experience some kind of mood instability in the first weeks postpartum. One minute you feel elated. The next you feel weepy. You get impatient. You get irritable. Yet feel fat and out of shape. You can't bear to look at yourself in the mirror. You don't seem to be able to control your moods.

Giving birth and crossing over to parenthood is a challenging and emotional time. The first few weeks and months, and even years, are a period of readjustment for both you and the baby. It's a myth that the baby blues only last a week or so after delivery. If you were used to routine, if you were used to freedom, if you were used to time alone, your whole world changes. Your baby will leave no part of your life untouched.

It's easy to feel overwhelmed as your routine changes and your new responsibilities and a demanding baby take over your life. You might begin to feel a little low. The event so anticipated has left you emotionally exhausted. At no other time in your life will you lose as much weight in so short a time. At no other time will hormone levels drop so dramatically. It took your body nine months to prepare for childbirth, and in about six weeks your body systems race to undo all that. There is also incredible fatigue to battle with. Labor and delivery is exhausting. Small wonder you probably feel exhausted. You are also sleep deprived.

Some of the emotions you experience may be bizarre. You might have weird dreams. You might wonder why on earth you ever had a baby at all. You might suddenly burst into tears. This is perfectly normal. Expect to feel a little strange for the first six weeks. Give your hormones and your life a chance to settle down. Rest as much as you can. Don't try to do everything yourself. Let your partner, your family, your friends help you and talk to them about how you are feeling.

Postpartum Depression and Weight Gain

Weight gain could be a trigger for postpartum depression (PPD), but it is a trigger and nothing more. PPD is a serious mood disorder that strikes about 10 percent of new mothers. "True postpartum depression is due to a chemical imbalance in the brain that is aggravated by a drop in pregnancy hormones postpartum and the stress of motherhood" (Dr. Jacobs).

In contrast to the baby blues, which strikes within days of birth, PPD strikes a little later. It usually happens about two weeks after delivery and can last for months. There could be insomnia, aversion to the baby, fear of harming the baby, loss of interest in your life.

Researchers believe that in addition to the hormonal shifts taking place, women who suffer from serious mood disorders after pregnancy have one or more biological and/or psychosocial vulnerabilities to the condition:

- There could be a prior history of depression
- There could be a family history of depression
- There could be serious hormonal problems
- Stressful events might happen at the same time, such as a death in the family, or a move
- There could be a complication with the pregnancy
- There might be some underlying disease or illness

If you think that you have something far more serious than the baby blues, see your doctor immediately. If you can't eat, sleep, or feel hopeless or out of control in any way, this is not normal. You need help. Prolonged maternal depression is dangerous for you and for baby. It is an illness. Don't be put off by people telling you it's just the baby blues. It isn't. There are times when you just can't snap out of depression. PPD can be very successfully treated with counseling and, if needed, medication. Try to join a support group in your area. If you can't find one in your area, get a referral from Depression After Delivery (DAD) at (800) 944-4773 or write to P.O. Box 1282, Morrisville, PA 19067.

Body Image Anxiety

What I'm talking about in this chapter, however, is not the "baby blues" that many, but not all, women suffer. I'm not talking about postpartum depression, either. I'm talking about a general dissatisfaction women have with their bodies that lingers on several months after baby is born.

As women often have difficulty separating what we are from what we look like, it is hardly surprising if you feel a little despondent after baby is born, you might blame those feelings on how out of shape you think you look. You might think that once you get your body back, all your insecurities will go away. Managing your weight is something positive you can do for yourself, but if you think that once you get down to a certain weight you will feel positive about your life again, you are very wrong. Your body and your life change with a baby. If you can't accept that, you will feel "heavy with child" whether you get to your target weight or not.

All too often, body image anxiety can become a way of coping with or avoiding other issues in your life. Like it or not, motherhood brings with it new responsibilities and pressures. You will be challenged as never before.

Let's take a look at some of the common feelings new moms often have to face.

You might feel that your baby gets all the attention now and nobody is interested in you anymore. "The pregnant princess has become the postpartum peasant....With one wave of the obstetrician's wand....you've done a reverse Cinderella." (Eisenberg, Murkoff, and Hathaway, *What to Expect When You're Expecting*, Workman, 1996, p. 547) It's natural to feel a little left out.

If you had a C section, you could have feelings of anxiety, disappointment, and inadequacy to deal with. You may have looked forward to a vaginal birth. You could still have discomfort from the surgery.

You might miss being pregnant. This is strange but true. Many women I talked to missed the unique bonding of pregnancy, the time when your baby was a part of you.

If this was your last pregnancy, this might make you sad. And if your pregnancy wasn't planned, you might feel guilty. Your relationship with your partner may not be all that you want it to be. If you don't have a partner, you may miss sharing your child with someone you love.

Perhaps you were so involved with your pregnancy that you forgot that there is life beyond. Suddenly you are on your own. You might find that it doesn't all come naturally to you. You may be anxious about your parenting skills. You may feel inadequate. Everything you do for baby seems to be wrong. You may have very little support from family and friends, or you could feel lonely if all your friends are not interested in babies. On the other hand, you could be depressed about family and friends who try to interfere too much.

Perhaps you had unrealistic expectations about motherhood. It is not going to make all your other problems go away. Life goes on. You may feel guilty that you don't enjoy being a mother as much as you thought you would. You may feel guilty for wanting time to yourself. Or you could have become so absorbed in motherhood you have no time or interest for anything else. You might worry that you can't seem to bond with your baby. You may find that you miss opportunities at work. You may have strong feelings of guilt if you have gone back to work, or regret if you have not. You may find it hard to cope financially.

You may miss the old you. Those carefree days in the past when you could go out at a moment's notice. When you could concentrate on your career, go out to dinner when you wanted, go to the movies when you wanted. You may miss intimate time with your partner, you used to do so many things together. Now there are always three of you. Your life has become one big juggling act. You never have time to do anything well.

You may even have had a history of body image problems before. More often than not, if a woman has obsessed about her weight before baby, she is likely to obsess about it after baby, too. If the tendency is there, pregnancy won't always make it go away.

Managing your weight is not the magic answer to these kinds of issues. If you have problems coming to terms with body changes, if your weight is spiraling our of control, if you are still dissatisfied with your body, the best thing to do is to take the focus from your weight to other areas of your life. There is so much more to life than the bathroom scales. Your beautiful baby, for one thing. Emphasis needs to be shifted from weight to the incredible transformation that has taken place in your life. You need to give yourself time to adjust. To recreate your life again. You need to understand that the old rules don't apply anymore. You have changed. You have become a mom. You can either view your new responsibilities as burdens or as incredible opportunities to make your life more fulfilled and enriched.

One of the ways women can do this is, as Christiane Northrup writes in *Women's Bodies, Women's Wisdom* (Bantam, 1995, p. 427) to "mother ourselves." Children are demanding. You need energy to raise them to be healthy and happy. It is very hard all by yourself to meet their demands without having some time for your own adult needs. You need to learn to take care of yourself. If you are happy and fulfilled, your baby will be, too. Talk to others. Ask for advice. Get active. Get all your nutrients. Try to cultivate a more healthy body image. Make time for yourself. Pamper yourself a little. You deserve it.

Northrup's advice is sound. New moms need to take better care of themselves. We also need to stop being so hard on ourselves. Constant self-sacrifice, trying to be the perfect mom, is not a "healthy path to motherhood." Constant self-criticism, trying to have the perfect body, is not a healthy and positive way to live.

And if you don't feel that bond developing with your baby, be patient. It will happen one day. Give yourself time. I loved my baby, but I felt disappointed. I didn't feel overwhelming love. I watched other mothers. I saw their faces transform with love whenever they looked at their baby. My face only ever seemed to look anxious. What was wrong with me?

Then one morning when my baby was seven months old, he reached out to give me a hug. Everything changed that day. An overwhelming joy and love for this little person filled my heart. I knew it would never go away.

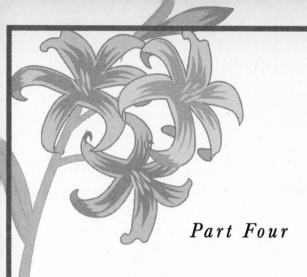

Part Four

Partners and Your Changing Body

What's the difference between a nine-month pregnant woman and a Playboy centerfold? Nothing, if the pregnant woman's partner knows what's good for them.

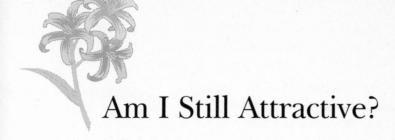

Am I Still Attractive?

DO THEY REALLY LIKE US WHEN WE ARE BIG-BREASTED AND PREGNANT? What do they think of those large stomachs? I asked a few partners to give me their honest opinion. Here's what some of them said. (Bear in mind, though, that every partner is an individual and will react to your changing body in his or her own way.)

"She got me excited when she was pregnant. I liked how she looked. She's got a soft stomach after the baby. I like that, too. She'll always be beautiful to me, however she looks." Michael, age 45, father of one

"In the first four months of her pregnancy she looked really sexy. But she has not lost as much weight as she hoped since delivery. It's making her unhappy. That's why I want her to lose it. I want her to be happier." James, age 40, father of three

"Her appearance didn't bother me. What did bother me were her mood swings. She always seemed to be on edge. She's working really hard to get rid of the excess weight—too hard, I think. I wish she would slow down a bit. She looks fine to me. You know it really makes me think twice about having another one. I don't want us to drift even further apart." Patrick, age 38, father of one

"Her body was different, but beautiful. I was fascinated by all the changes. I like her big breasts and stomach. Her swollen hands and feet and constant backache made things a

149

little difficult at times. After the baby she lost a lot of weight. She still needs to work on her stomach, though, to get back to where she was." Christopher, age 30, father of two

"She got huge when she was pregnant. We both knew it would be a struggle to lose the weight afterwards. It's going to take a lot of exercise and dieting for her to get back in shape. I only mind for her. I want her to feel good. She knows I love her whatever she looks like." Michelle, age 39, mother of one

"It's important to me that my wife gets back in shape. I would like to see her lose some weight. It makes her look younger and more sexy. She's also much happier when she is slimmer." Robin, age 43, father of two

"I was into the experience from day one. I felt that it brought us closer together. Her appearance was just part of that experience. It varied throughout her pregnancy, but even when she was at her heaviest there were moments of hilarity that somehow took away the moments of tension." Ray, age 48, father of one.

Weight Gain and Relationships

Many of us might worry about how our changing bodies will affect our relationships. We may not feel so sexual anymore. We might worry that our partners will lose interest in us physically as our bodies change. We often assume that when we lose our waistline we instantly become unattractive. From my interviews with the partners of pregnant women, this was not usually the case. Partners are far more accepting and appreciative of bodily change than is often thought. What did come across, however, from talking to moms-to-be and new moms was that when a woman feels unattractive, she finds it hard to imagine that anyone else can find her attractive. There is often so much anxiety that even a compliment can be turned into something negative.

During pregnancy and childbirth, a woman's changing body can trigger relationship problems. Sadly, some relationships do end. Unable to accept how a woman looks, the partner attempts to resolve stress by either distancing him- or herself from the relationship or having an affair with someone else. In almost all cases, though, mom's appearance is not the real issue. It becomes an excuse to mask other conflicts and tensions within the relationship.

Then there are women who become obsessive about their bodies because they fear that their partners will leave them if they gain weight. This is terrible for self-esteem. It's as dysfunctional as the woman who turns to food for comfort when she feels insecure and gains far too much weight, even though she knows this is hurting both herself and her partner.

I talked to many pregnant and postpartum mothers and it was clear that changes in their appearance did affect their relationship in a number of ways. Some found that it made the bond between them stronger. Others were more anxious. Whatever the reaction of partners, though, there was agreement on one thing. Every mother needed to feel that she was still desirable. She needed to know that her partner still enjoyed and accepted her new body. For most of us, this was the single most important thing our partners could do for us.

And the best way to get this kind of appreciation it seems is to tell your partner how you feel about your body. "Clearly express to your partner how important it is he or she appreciate your body," writes Jennifer Louden in *The Pregnant Woman's Comfort Book* (Harper San Francisco, 1995, p. 62).

If your partner makes negative comments, Louden encourages you to use them as an opportunity for discussion. This is good advice. You and your partner should discuss what your body is going through. If your partner feels nervous about your pregnant body, talk about it. If postpartum weight gain is bothering your partner, talk about it. If you don't, resentment, anger, and frustration will creep in. You need to find out if your partner is concerned about your health and wants what is best for you, or if there are other issues involved that have nothing to do with how much you weigh and more to do with a relationship that is in crisis. (Needless to say, any person who is deliberately hurtful about your weight gain is not acting in your best interests.)

Telling our partners how much we need them to appreciate our bodies is key, but far too few women make this step. We keep our weight anxiety a big, shameful secret. Many partners probably have no idea that this is such a sensitive area. Innocent comments can upset us.

Too often we assume that we aren't attractive anymore without even asking. We forget that our partners might be having anxieties of their own. If we don't talk to each other, the result is tears and confusion.

What about Sex During Pregnancy?

You may have read that, unless yours is a high-risk pregnancy, you can have sex right up to the day of delivery. But would you want to?

Few of the women I talked to could honestly say that pregnancy had not affected their sex life until the last few weeks. Some women may feel intensely erotic when pregnant, but most of us won't and have to make do with the occasional moment of passion until life returns to some semblance of normality. Sexual interest seemed to peak for most couples in the second trimester, but for others it did not peak at all. Most confessed that during pregnancy sex was far less frequent. There's the physical discomfort for a start. Nausea, headache, an expanding belly, and a weak bladder do not spell a sexual turn-on. These discomforts may leave you feeling very vulnerable.

Many couples worried about whether sex was safe or not. The answer is simple. Sex is safe during pregnancy. It will not bring on premature labor. The only time you need to be concerned is if there is a history of first trimester miscarriage or premature labor, if unexplained bleeding occurs, if multiple fetuses are carried, if waters have broken, or if there are complications to your pregnancy and your doctor advises against intercourse. In all other cases, sex during pregnancy is not only safe but desirable, especially if the emphasis is on lovemaking and strengthening your relationship.

Whether sex is better than ever, just uncomfortable, or almost nonexistent during your pregnancy, you will find that sexual relations between you and your partner will alter in some way. This is normal. If sex is less frequent than before, it can be just as rewarding if the emphasis shifts to quality rather than quantity. If sex feels less enjoyable, both you and your partner can keep your sexual relationship strong by talking about and trying to understand the many changes pregnancy brings. Both you and your partner have to adjust not only to your changing body, but to the idea that you are no longer lovers but parents. There is real hope that in time these changes will replace any sexual anxieties you may have with excitement and satisfaction.

Everyone in Your Life Has to Adjust to the New You

Once you get pregnant, you have to come to terms with the fact that you are not the only one who is going to have mixed feelings about your body. This is especially the case if staying in shape and being thin was your lifestyle. Partners, friends, and family may feel nervous, even afraid, of the changes they see happening to you in so short a space of time. They may need time to adjust. This does not mean that you are not loved anymore. The people in your life are just finding the change hard to accept. Be patient. Just as you need time, they do too. Remind yourself that nothing stays the same forever. Life moves on, and true friendships and partnerships will survive these changes.

17

Is There Sex after Birth?

THE WHOLE EXPERIENCE OF CHILDBIRTH MIGHT MAKE YOU FEEL BETTER about your body—more feminine and erotic. You may find it easier to get aroused because of improved circulation in the pelvic area. Having a baby could bring you closer to your partner than ever before, and sex is a way to express your love and bonding.

> "I couldn't wait to dispel the cold sterile hospital feel," says Rachel, age 30, "with some physical closeness with my husband. My doctor told me to wait, but we had sex three weeks after I gave birth."

If you are ready and willing for sex, your doctor will probably advise that you wait six weeks until the first postpartum checkup. There is a reason for this. You should not have sex until your cervix is properly closed. If you do, bacteria might enter into the uterus. It is important that the vagina and perineal tissues be healed, too. The end of bleeding in the weeks following birth usually signals that your uterus and cervix have recovered.

If having a baby has enhanced your sex life, this is fantastic. You are in the minority, though. Most of us find ourselves wondering if there is sex after birth.

What's Wrong with Me?

> "It took me about a year to feel comfortable with sex again."

"At six months postpartum I still didn't want my husband to see me naked."

"I just wasn't interested in sex for the first few months."

We probably have read about or talked to a woman who resumed sexual intercourse at about three weeks, but studies show that most of us feel as much like sex after having a baby as having our wisdom teeth out.

Managing your weight will help you feel better about your body and your sexuality, but problems with arousal are a common occurrence after birth. In a 1989 St. Paul, Minnesota, study, research on women's health in the postpartum period found that nearly half were still not comfortable with intercourse at three months for a variety of reasons. A fifth still had problems after a year. The problem isn't discussed much, though, which can make a woman feel she is the only one or that there is something wrong with her.

Feeling anxious about how you look is perhaps one reason why most women do not resume sex right away, or that when they do it is less frequent than before. Extra fat on your hips and thighs, a soft belly, heavy breasts, and other postpartum discomforts, as well as sensitivity about your scar if you had a C section and embarrassment about the extra pounds gained, can all lead to inhibitions for either or both parties. One woman told me that at eight months postpartum, and still twenty pounds over her prepregnancy weight, her husband told her she didn't look as good as before. After that, she never let him see her naked and only wanted to have sex in the dark.

But many other factors may also be contributing to lower libido after birth.

FEELING DRY

Normally, during sex the hormone estrogen lubricates your vagina. But in the early months after giving birth estrogen levels are low. You may not lubricate easily. Sex could be feel painful and dry for both you and your partner. Vaginal dryness goes away when estrogen levels return to normal. This might take longer if you are breastfeeding. Many experts believe that when you are nursing, sexual desire is actually suppressed by the hormone prolactin. Other experts disagree, but studies show that lack of desire for sex when nursing is not uncommon.

While you are feeling dry, you can make sex more comfortable by giving yourself more time to get aroused. Spend more time playing with each other prior to intercourse, or use a lubricant such as KY jelly or a cream for your vagina to make intercourse more pleasurable.

LOOSE VAGINA

Your vaginal opening might be looser than it was prepregnancy, making intercourse less pleasurable for you and your partner. Tightening up the pelvic area with kegels and losing weight will help. (See Chapter Twenty-Three for more information about kegels.)

SORE PERINEUM

If you had an episiotomy, this can take longer than six weeks to heal. When your doctor says you are healed, this means only that the early stage of healing is complete. The scar tissue left by the incision will still be tender for about six months, and sex could be painful while it heals. Strengthening your pelvic floor muscles and massaging the area with an estrogen cream can speed recovery.

TENDER AND LEAKING BREASTS

If you are breastfeeding, your breasts might become engorged when you have sex. Right in the middle of sex you could also start leaking all over your partner. (The hormone oxytocin, released during orgasm, is also responsible for the letdown of milk reflex.) Sex is by nature a juicy business, and you might find this increases your pleasure. But if you don't relish the idea of heavy, leaking breasts, or your partner sucking your breasts when you have been nursing all day, you can make yourself feel more comfortable by wearing a bra during sex or having sex when your breasts aren't too full. You might treat yourself to a sexy-looking bra and make putting it on part of your erotic play!

CESAREAN INCISION

Just like an episiotomy, a cesarean section scar may take longer than six weeks to heal. Soreness and pain may take up to a year to go away. You will have to work on finding a position with your partner that is comfortable. With a sore abdomen and possibly a dry vagina, sex may not be as pleasurable as it could be for a while.

FEELING TOO TIRED

When your doctor tells you at your six-week checkup that you can have sex again, you might wonder where on earth you are going to get the energy. Fatigue could have become a part of your life. The new responsibility of a baby can be exhausting in the early months, and if you do have any free time, you might prefer sleep to sex.

Rather than having sex because you feel you ought to, it is far better to show your affection in other ways. Cuddling can be very satisfying, as can spending more time together and talking about how you feel. In this way you can grow close again. The closer you feel, the more likely it is that sex will follow as an expression of your closeness.

JUST NOT IN THE MOOD

Loss of libido after having a baby is common. You may not feel the same level of arousal for your partner as you did before. Just because sex could be low on your list of priorities doesn't mean that you don't love your partner anymore. Physical discomfort could explain why you feel the way you do, but psychological as well as physical factors contribute to diminished arousal after birth. Here's what some new moms said about sex at six months postpartum.

"My body has been prodded and poked for nine months. I don't see myself sexually at the moment."

"I feel like my body has been invaded and taken over. I just want time to myself."

"I love being a mom. It's so hard to transform into a sexual partner after being in mom mode all day."

"I'm finding it hard to feel close to my boyfriend. His life has not changed at all. But my body, my lifestyle, everything about me has changed."

"My husband says he finds it difficult to have sex with me after watching me give birth."

"I had a difficult labor and delivery. I really don't want to get pregnant again."

"In the early months I worried that I might get an infection."

"I get all the love and hugs I need from my baby."

"I get a lot of satisfaction and comfort from nursing."

"I can't relax. I always think my baby might cry or need something when I try to have sex."

"I really don't like my body. I feel overweight and flabby. I just don't have the confidence for sex right now."

You and your partner need to both give each other time to adjust emotionally to all the changes that have taken place in so short a space of time. Talking to each other about how you feel is often the best remedy. If this doesn't help, seeking guidance from a counselor might.

Hormonal Imbalance

Weight may be a critical factor as far as loss of sex drive is concerned, but there may also be other factors involved. For instance, hormonal imbalance. There are massive hormonal shifts after pregnancy and delivery, and hormonal imbalance is associated with low sex drive. An imbalance in your estrogen and progesterone levels can affect you in many ways, including sexually. Studies also show that if testosterone or DHEA levels are too low, this could have a profound effect on your libido.

So far, doctors don't really understand the role of testosterone and DHEA and how they determine your sex drive, but you could ask your doctor to do a blood test of serum free testosterone and serum DHEA. If these are low, prescribing testosterone might help. Testosterone cream applied to the genital area is another method. DHEA is now available over the counter but make sure you check with your doctor for a dosage that is right for you.

Dealing with the Postpartum Sexual Slump

If you find you have no interest at all in sex a year postpartum and it is starting to affect your relationship, you should think about consulting your doctor to determine the cause.

You might prefer to seek counseling from a skilled sexual therapist. This can often be helpful. As far as aphrodisiacs are concerned, certain natural, plant, or nutritional remedies for libido can work, but they are not always reliable. Making sure you get sufficient B vitamins might help. The herbs ginseng and damiana could have a positive effect, as could adrenal extracts and DHEA. Homeopathic remedies for loss of sex drive like Sepia, Natrum mur, and phosphoric acid work for some women. Alternative remedies such as acupuncture might also prove useful.

Don't make the mistake of assuming that you won't enjoy sex again. Things will return to normal eventually. You may have to wait until your hormones have returned to their prepregnancy state and you feel more confident about your body again, but in time you will feel sexual again. The post partum sexual slump is not forever. And during this period the chances are that you will have grown closer in other ways. After all, you and your partner have the most incredible bond. You have created the miracle of new life together.

In the meantime, there are many ways you can deal with sexual problems after birth. Talking to your partner about sex, finding other ways to express your love, experimenting with positions, using artificial lubrication, finding time to be alone together, having sex when you can and not just at bedtime, emphasizing quality not quantity— these can all help. Eating right, exercising, tightening your vagina with kegels, and improving your body image will certainly improve things, too. But remember—having satisfying sex after birth is affected not just by the physical, but by the psychological. Your body may have healed, but your emotions may take far longer to sort themselves out.

Give yourself and your partner time to ease back into sex. Your partner may also have had a significant postpartum sexual slump, too. He or she might have emotional and physical issues to deal with as well. They might have been put off by the experience of watching the birth, of seeing you nurse, of watching your body change so dramatically in the last nine months, of seeing you in the new role of mother. They may be worried about hurting you or even have body image problems themselves.

As the next Chapter shows, we often tend to forget that our partners have just as much adjusting to the new role of parent to do as we do, so we will look at that next.

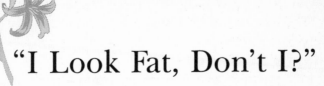

18

"I Look Fat, Don't I?"

BY RAY CHEUNG

I LOOK FAT, DON'T I?

Never answer that question directly.

As soon as my wife was pregnant she told me she looked huge. I couldn't see any difference. She said I must be blind. So when she did put on a few pounds I told her she looked heavier. (When you're pregnant you've got to put on weight, right? It's a sign things are going well, isn't it?) I thought this would reassure her. Big mistake. I soon learned that this was the worst possible thing I could do. She was in a bad mood all week.

The advice Frank Munegeam gives in *A Guy's Guide to Pregnancy* (Beyond Words, 1998, p. 41) is solid. "Most of the time telling the truth in relationships is a good thing. During pregnancy, however, some of the time tested rules of communication—like being honest—don't always apply." Munegeam advises men to answer in the negative if their pregnant partners ask if they are showing or if they look heavy and the affirmative if they ask whether they look attractive,

Munegeam is right when he says "women take weight gain more personally than men." I never fully realized this until my wife got pregnant. I could sense that her changing shape caused her anxiety. She felt uncomfortable in maternity clothes. She worried that she wouldn't lose all the weight postpartum. She thought being pregnant would change my feelings for her. It all seemed illogical to me. Of course she was going to gain weight. The baby had to come from somewhere.

Deep down I think my wife knew she was being illogical. Reading between the lines, I realized that what she really wanted to know was whether I still found her desirable. To be perfectly honest, I did. The

------ 161 ------

last month or two was a little more difficult. Her belly just dominated everything. I didn't tell her, though. Pregnancy is not a permanent state. I reassured her as best I could.

Constantly Reassure

The advice I give to partners of pregnant women is to reassure them constantly of your affection. It works wonders. You may as well get in good practice. Your partner's weight loss postpartum is going to be just as sensitive a topic as her weight gain during pregnancy. She'll need to be reassured about that, too. She needs to know that you still find her attractive after the baby. Usually with time she'll lose most of the weight, but don't bully her if her body changes a little. After all, she's been through a lot.

A *Fit Pregnancy* article entitled "Pregnant Pas" (Spring 1998, p. 40), in their regular and highly readable "birth of a father" series, was right on the ball. The author, Paul Feldman, described a day spent with a water-weighted vest with two seven-pound lead balls that represent fetal limbs and a six-pound weight to put pressure on the bladder. This is in fact a "Pregnancy Simulator" marketed by Birthways, Inc., of Vashon Island, Washington, to help partners understand how it really feels to be pregnant. "At full weight I had difficulty breathing, walking around and relieving myself. The belly also guaranteed a flood of jokes," writes Feldman.

So give your partner a break. It seems obvious that pregnancy and childbirth are exhausting and demanding experiences. You don't really need to go so far as to wear a simulator to appreciate the tremendous physical and emotional changes your partner is going through. Tell her you still find her attractive. Let her have some time for herself so that she can come back refreshed and feeling better about herself and her body. Listen to her. Give her some leeway for moodiness. Make sure you really are an equal partner in child care. Those early bonds with your child are the strongest.

Having a baby in your life is a period of great readjustment for both you and her. You might be stressed or unhappy about your weight as well, so for the time being give yourself as well as mom a break. You have both been through a lot. Wait until you are both emotionally and physically ready before you begin a weight management program.

Childbirth has given me a profound new respect for my partner's strength and energy. How remarkable the female body is! The bond between us has grown stronger. As long as she is healthy and happy, it really is immaterial to me whether or not she returns to her prepregnancy weight. I think most fathers and partners would feel the same.

But trying to convince my wife that I'm telling the truth when I say I still find her attractive when she has asked me for the hundredth time, "I look fat don't I?" is going to be as challenging as getting back in shape myself.

Why do I need to get back in shape? Well, here's my experience.

How I Experienced Pregnancy and Postpartum

As soon as we decided to make a baby, I made the decision to get really fit. I started to jog, swim, run, and lift weights regularly. After six months, my wife was still not pregnant and I was convinced something was wrong with me. I started to exercise even more and get even fitter.

Then came that memorable day when she told me I was going to be a dad. I was thrilled. We had done it. Almost immediately, though, I started to worry if the baby would be healthy and if my wife would cope. I also wondered how much it would all cost.

During the first trimester it wasn't that easy to get excited yet. My wife was sick all the time. Sex was nonexistent. I went to a few of her prenatal exams, but I admit I felt out of place. It was incredible seeing the heartbeat, but my baby-to-be looked like a tadpole, so I found it hard to get emotionally involved. I concentrated on eating healthily and exercising regularly, as I wanted to be fit when I became a dad. I made sure my wife took her vitamins. Pregnancy made her forgetful. It also made her a little too fond of chocolate. For the baby-to-be's sake, I asked her to cut down.

We changed doctors in the second trimester. This one actually noticed me at the prenatal exams and didn't treat me like a piece of furniture. I think it was about now that I began to feel a bit left out. My wife seemed very preoccupied with the baby-to-be, especially when she could feel it move. In some ways I was relieved as she seemed less dependent on me. It also gave me a chance to watch what I wanted on TV while she slept on the sofa. She wanted to have sex again in this trimester. Although it was good to be intimate again, I was more worried about the baby than she was. I was scared I might squash it.

The third trimester wasn't so much fun. We didn't do as much together as she got bigger. We stopped our daily runs and my fitness levels declined. I never knew what to say to her. Some days everything I said or did was wrong. Sex was off the agenda again. She was just too big. She tossed and turned a lot at night and had difficulty sleeping. There were lots of midnight snacks. She started to crave calamari. We ate a lot of calamari. I went up a trouser size.

I started to buy things for the nursery in the last month. It was much more expensive than I thought. People at work were generous with a fantastic baby shower. They all asked how my wife was. This sounds a little pathetic, but I wished that just once they had asked how I was coping. She got very worried about having to have a C section when the doctor said the baby-to-be had a big head. She thought it wouldn't be the same as a vaginal birth. I had no special yearning to see my baby born in the traditional way, so I tried to reassure her. Indeed, I thought a C section would be incredible to watch, and at least I wouldn't have to put into practice all those coaching tips I had learned at prenatal classes.

I needed that advice from the prenatal classes, though, when it came to delivery. I also wished I had stayed in shape in the last few months. Two days without food and sleep—you can't call hospital food "food." I was shattered. I just wish she had gone for the epidural earlier. I would have. Things were so much more relaxed when she finally got her shot. I think on the whole I was a good coach, though. In the end there was no C section. I wasn't squeamish at all when the baby came out. It was a thrilling experience. I became a dad. Wow! A beautiful baby boy.

The first week postpartum is a bit of a blur. I hated how I looked in the hospital photos—dark circles under my eyes, and the camera angle made me look as if I was getting a pot belly.

As the weeks passed, the baby screamed more and more. I tried to make fitness a priority—after all, I couldn't afford to be ill now—but all too often it became the last priority. My wife seemed a bit sad for a month or so. I think she was just a bit overwhelmed. At least I could go back to work and have a sense of order and routine again. She couldn't.

At six weeks postpartum my wife began to look better. I looked worse. I was putting on weight. Neither of us felt comfortable about sex yet. By the time the baby finally got to sleep, there just wasn't any energy left. I hoped that in a few months I would feel better, but at six months postpartum I was still tired. At six months I also wondered where all my money had gone. I'd never thought having a baby was so expensive. The makers of formula must be making a fortune. And why does my wife insist on buying three of everything? Three strollers. Three car seats.

The days seemed to rush by. We finally got back to regular sex, but like everything else it is rushed. When my son was seven months I decided to buy trousers a size bigger and put the smaller ones away. My wife got a bit upset and wanted me to exercise more, but with work, travel for work, financial planning, and the baby, when am I going to find the time to work on my waistline?

And now at almost one year postpartum I am still constantly tired. Finances seem to have stabilized a bit, though. I have gained fifteen pounds since the baby was born. Think it looks good on me, though. I look mature, solid, dependable. Like a father should look. None of the other fathers at work exercise. My wife wants me to exercise, though, so maybe when things calm down a little at work (it's hectic at the moment), I'll get back into an exercise routine.

We must be crazy. We are thinking about having another one. How much will two of them cost?

Couvade Syndrome

In one of the many pregnancy books my wife gave me to read (why do they have to be at least 500 pages long?), there was a short chapter addressed to partners. It was informative, but what fascinated me was a tiny paragraph about a little-known disorder known as couvade syndrome.

"Couvade syndrome is well known by anthropologists, and had been described primarily in 'primitive cultures," writes Shapiro in *When Men Are Pregnant* (Delta, 1987, p. 82). There are varying degrees of couvade syndrome, and symptoms usually begin at the end of the first trimester right up until delivery. The word comes from the

French "to latch." Basically, a man starts to imitate many of the pregnancy symptoms his wife is experiencing—nausea, weight gain, food cravings, constipation, leg cramps, fatigue, and mood swings. There are many theories to explain couvade, and they include jealousy, feeling left out, identification with your wife, sympathy for your wife, guilt (after all, you put your wife in this position!), and anxiety about coping with your wife's mood swings and becoming a father.

Shapiro goes on to state that a great deal of recent evidence indicates that many men in modern cultures do experience pregnancy-like symptoms during the expectant period. In fact, *What to Expect When You're Expecting* (Eisenberg, Murkoff, and Hathaway, Workman, 1996, p. 415) estimates that up to 65 percent of men apparently suffer from this syndrome when their wives are pregnant. If this is so, why do we hear so little about it? For a very unfair reason. Partners are not supposed to get ill when their wives are pregnant.

Unfortunately, the condition is often misdiagnosed as something else, because when men go and see a doctor they rarely think to mention that their wives are pregnant. Complaining about your health when your wife is pregnant is taboo. If a man "comes out" with couvade syndrome, he is often ridiculed. So he suffers in silence.

A Woman's Partner Has Needs, Too

"In all my years as a therapist I have never seen a male client whose appearance was his primary concern." (Mary Pipher, *Hunger Pains*, Ballantine, 1995, p. 15)

Men don't have the same body image problems as women do. We discuss our bodies in different ways. We don't tend to blame our problems on our appearance.

I look at myself realistically. I don't think I am fatter than I am.

When I try on a new suit, I look at the suit. I don't criticize my body.

When my stock prices fall, I don't blame it on my weight.

When a relationship does not work, I don't blame my weight.

When clothes don't fit, I try another size.

I really don't worry that much about how I look.

But this was all before my wife got pregnant. These past two years I have been anxious about my weight and my health on many occasions.

The advice I give to pregnant women everywhere is, spare a thought for your partners. Pregnancy is a life-changing experience for them as well. You might not be the only one worried about your weight. Partners and "fathers are entitled to a few worries of their own and to some very special reassurance, not only during the pregnancy and the birth but in the post partum period as well," write the experts in *What to Expect When You're Expecting* (Eisenberg, Murkoff, and Hathaway, Workman, 1996, p. 412).

Your partner may not get couvade, but rare is the person who never took a sick day during their partner's pregnancy. It's a stressful time for us, too. And don't jump to the conclusion that if your partner does not gain weight or feel nausea for you, this means he or she has less sympathy for you. Remember, we all react differently to pressure and cope with it in different ways.

For me, I coped with the stress by keeping busy and by getting really fit when she was pregnant. I felt terrific during most of the pregnancy. I exercised. I ate well. I used to drive my wife crazy with my obsession with healthy eating for the baby. I nagged her when she didn't take her vitamins. I encouraged her to exercise. I built things around the house. I got the nursery ready. Towards the end I got very tired. It seemed like she had been pregnant forever. But on the whole I felt great.

Postpartum was a different story. I'm beginning to think I may be suffering from some kind of post-couvade syndrome. Sympathy symptoms for my wife postpartum. Now we've had the baby, we seem to be growing more alike each day.

Both of us are tired. Apparently, it takes most couples about two years to feel on top of things again and to lose that tired feeling. We both get moody—probably because we are both tired. And we're not at our prepregnancy weights. Perhaps that's something to do with the coffee and cakes we enjoy so much. But that's looking on the down side. On the up side, we are healthy, happy, and in love. We are a family.

Part Five

Weight Management After Baby

It's not what babies do to your body,
but what they do to your life.

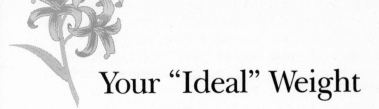

19

Your "Ideal" Weight

"I've got my six-week checkup tomorrow and I'm nowhere near my ideal weight."

"I've still got about seven pounds to lose to get to my ideal weight"

Most of us feel less anxious if we are within recommended ideal weight ranges for our height. But, as we saw in Part Two, height and weight charts give you only a vague idea of your ideal weight for your height. They are typically based on mortality data from people who buy life insurance, not disease and mortality statistics from the general population. These charts do not address the biological variability between women. How different our builds are. How our weight can fluctuate on a daily basis and with the seasons throughout the year.

One of the best things you can do when trying to manage your weight postpartum is to stop thinking about weight and concentrate on how your body feels. Trust that it knows what your natural weight should be. Motherhood offers you a wonderful opportunity to escape from what Christiane Northrup describes in *Women's Bodies, Women's Wisdom* (Bantam, 1995, p. 576) as the "diet mentality"—when the number you read on the scales determines whether you have a good or a bad day and stands between you and how you experience your life.

Throw Away the Scales

When you start to eat for weight loss, you initially lose water and glycogen from your muscles. The scales give you an encouragement.

You lose a few pounds. But the next week, when you weigh yourself, you haven't lost any more. The same thing happens the following week. You get less motivated. Your diet isn't working. You give up.

The reason you have stopped losing weight is because your body, fearing starvation, starts to cling to its fat stores. In fact, this is the most important time to keep eating healthily. You are close to losing fat, but it's going to take time. That's why staying away from the scales is important. They can demoralize you when you don't "see" any progress.

Scales do not help you lose weight. They give unreliable and misleading information. Every day your weight fluctuates. The scales don't tell you about emotional weight gain, either, when you have been eating poorly because you are tired or sad. "Don't rely on the scale to determine if you're successful or to provide you with a sense of self accomplishment," writes Colleen Sunder Meyer. "If you want to gain control over your eating and your body weight, get rid of the scale and listen to your own feelings. You can trust yourself" (*I Want My Body Back*, Perigee, 1995, p. 26).

The best advice I can give all moms struggling with post partum weight loss is to keep away from scales of any kind until the number you read on the scales has lost its power to determine whether you feel good or bad.

If you must have some kind of reference, a far better way to see if you are at a healthy weight is to ignore the weight charts and get your body fat tested. (Normal body fat measurement is 28 to 30 percent. Under 25 percent is fit and slender. Lower than 22 percent is too thin. Higher than 30 percent is too heavy.)

Change Your Body Image

"There comes a time to stop trying to change or hoping to change your body, and to start changing the way you feel about it," writes Jacqueline Shannon (*The New Mother's Body Book*, Contemporary Books, 1994, p. 230).

Being thin is not the same as being healthy, happy, and energized. While writing this book, I spoke to many moms about weight loss postpartum. Even those who had reached their prepregnancy weight were still uncomfortable with their bodies. They still wanted to lose a few more pounds. They still hated what they called their "ugly stretch marks," their "flabby butts," and "soggy stomachs." Women both thin and overweight expressed to me how heavy they felt and burdened down with anxiety about how they looked.

Having a baby offers us a real chance to come to terms with feelings of dissatisfaction about our bodies. There is a reason motherhood is such a great time to do this. It is a time of new beginnings and fresh starts. You are a role model now for your baby. You don't want your baby to have body image problems. You want your baby to have a positive body image. And that starts with you, if not celebrating your body, then at least respecting it.

Creating a positive body image is extremely hard if you have grown up being critical of your looks. Here are some tips that might get you started in the right direction:

- Have a good long think about why exactly you want to be thinner. Why is it so important to you?
- Do some research. In many cultures around the world, being thin is not considered attractive. In times past, too, the idea of beauty was far from thin, as we saw in Chapter Two.
- Listen to your body. Commit to trusting that it knows what it wants. Be honest about what you are eating. Recognize emotional eating when you are using food to avoid facing other issues in your life. Make sensible food choices. Eat when you are hungry. Stop when you are full.
- Exercise when you can. Not only will this improve body confidence; it will speed up your metabolism.
- Look after yourself. Give yourself the same love and respect you give your baby. Pamper yourself once in a while. You deserve it.
- If your weight is really making you depressed, try to seek professional help. You need guidance about how to change negative thought patterns, and a therapist might help. Call an eating disorder clinic at your hospital and ask for a referral. To keep you on track, you might consider joining a support group that deals with food, weight, and depression.

- Read some books on self-esteem and developing a healthy body image.
- Recognize that it is unnatural and unhealthy to be as thin as the models on the catwalks. They are not "real" women but fantasies created by the media.
- Understand that thinness does not equal attractiveness.
- Separate what you do from how you look.
- Focus on what you are good at. Put your energy into other things. Focus on other areas in your life.
- Think positively about your body. Focus on what you like. You are just as attractive as before, in a different way.
- Look into your baby's eyes. Doesn't that make everything seem worthwhile?

And finally, remember that change is inevitable. Even the most enthusiastic fitness routine, the most nutritious diet can't defeat Mother Nature. Every woman is going to face physical change over time—even women who have never breastfed or given birth. If you consider yourself unattractive, others may pick up on your drop in self-esteem and be more affected by your change in attitude than by any change in your body. If you have made peace with some of the effects of childbirth and have confidence in your body, you will probably look sexier and more attractive than you have ever been.

A positive body image makes any woman look attractive, regardless of how much she weighs and how many babies she has had or is having. Gaining this kind of body confidence starts with treating your body with respect. The next chapters will discuss reasons for slow weight loss, the effects of breastfeeding versus bottle-feeding, and finally, how you can treat your body with respect by eating healthily, exercising regularly, and reducing the amount of stress in your life.

20

Why Can't I Lose
This Baby Fat?

IT ALL SEEMS SO EASY WHEN YOU READ THE ARTICLES. BEAUTIFUL MOM
and baby laughing together, exercising together.

"Get your body back after baby."

"Working out with baby. The fastest way to get in shape."

"New baby, new body, new life. How to get it all together."

"Bounce back after baby."

"Shaping up after baby."

"Six weeks to shape up after baby."

"Life After Baby: Lose weight. Stay sane. A real life plan
for moms."

Then one morning you wake up and panic. It's six weeks since
baby was born.

Exercise—you must be joking. You haven't got the energy.
Sleep—you are constantly tired.
Time to yourself—you don't have it.
Getting things done when baby naps—your baby doesn't nap.
Diet—you are eating all the time.
Breastfeeding—you are constantly hungry.
Clothes—you are still wearing leggings and long sweaters.
Weight—you still have fifteen pounds to lose.

What went wrong? Why couldn't you be like those happy, thin moms in the magazines?

Nothing has gone wrong. You are normal. Being overweight several months postpartum is usual. Few, if any, moms get their figures back after six weeks, despite what the books say.

In her always hilarious *Girlfriends' Guide to Surviving the First Year of Motherhood* (Perigee, 1997, p. 141), which I highly recommend for its reassuring and irreverent tone, Vicki Iovine gives some sound advice about postpartum flab. "It's so depressing, I know, but it's normal. Why should we expect a condition that took us nine (ten) months to develop to disappear in a couple of weeks?"

The following might shed some light on the mystery of postpartum baby fat and at the same time offer some valuable advice.

Still Eating for Two

You might not be losing weight because you're still eating for two. When you were pregnant, you probably got used to eating lots of food. You were eating to supply your baby with all the nutrients he needed. Now you have to adjust your appetite and your mind to the fact that you are not eating for two anymore. Sometimes your hunger might be hard to control. But unless you want to look pregnant forever, you are going to have to change some old habits. The sooner you start really thinking about what you are eating, you can start to recognize when you are eating more than you really want, eating too fast, and eating more often than you really need. Slowly you can start replacing your old eating patterns with healthy new ones.

The Sacrificial Mom

Perhaps you're not losing those extra pounds because you're afraid it will harm your baby. Many new moms are so concerned that they give their baby adequate nutrients that their own health and appearance takes second place. This is especially so for breastfeeding moms.

Although dieting for weight loss while breastfeeding is not recommended, your aim should be to eat a healthy diet that stops you gaining any further weight. Remember, your health and appearance affect your self-esteem, and a lowered self-esteem is not good for either you or your baby. One of the best things you can do for your baby is take care of you. He needs a happy, healthy role model he can admire.

Did You Have Weight Management Problems Before and During Pregnancy?

Gaining the amount of weight recommended for your pregnancy and beginning your pregnancy at a normal weight are the best ways to avoid weight management problems postpartum. If you were significantly overweight before you got pregnant or gained a huge amount during your pregnancy, weight management will be much harder postpartum.

Have You Changed Your Approach to Diet and Exercise?

> "Once you have a baby...you'll be a changed person psychologically and biochemically. You'll be adjusting to a new baby, a new lifestyle, a new metabolism, and a new appetite." (Colleen Sundermeyer, *I Want My Body Back*, Perigee, 1998, p. 16)

Many women make the mistake of using diet and exercise routines that worked for them prepregnancy in the postpartum period. They get very disappointed when weight doesn't come off. There is a reason why this happens. Your body has gone through a tremendous change in a very short space of time. What worked in the past won't work any more. There are new rules to be learned. Your old self doesn't exist anymore. You are a mother now. You have different priorities. You have a different body, and you need to find new ways to work with it.

Body Awareness

Perhaps the body awareness you gained during pregnancy is slipping away. During pregnancy many women are more attuned to their body than ever before. You listen to the signals your body sends you. It's a shame that this often stops postpartum. We go back to poor eating habits once baby is born or we stop breastfeeding. We lose that body awareness. With poor body awareness, weight management problems are far more likely.

It is crucial for successful weight management postpartum that you carry the body awareness of pregnancy with you into motherhood. Your body just knew what to do when you were pregnant. That wisdom doesn't go away when baby is born. It's important that you keep listening to your postpartum body just as you did when you were pregnant. Trust your body. It really does know what is best for you.

Comparing Yourself with Others

> "My friend Rachel has gotten back to her prepregnancy weight already. I'm hardly eating. Why am I not losing weight, too?"

It really is pointless comparing yourself to someone else. You don't have the same lifestyle, biology, and metabolic rate as another woman. What works for her may not work for you. No two women are alike. That's why well-meaning advice or videos, books, and magazines that promote certain routines and diet plans postpartum may not work for you, however hard you try. They are not tailored to your needs, your body, and your lifestyle. The only body you should be focusing on right now in terms of weight management is your own. What works for your body won't work for someone else's. What's normal for you won't be normal for someone else. We are all different. We will all lose weight in different ways, too.

You need to appreciate how unique your body is. For weight management to be a success, you need to take into account everything about your unique life and your unique body. Understanding your uniqueness will help you create a postpartum weight loss plan that is right for you. Think about the following....

YOUR AGE

If you are in your teens or twenties, weight loss will be much easier than if you are older. Youth gives you the energy you need to lose those pounds. Physiologically, the twenties are the ideal time to have a baby, because miscarriage, infertility, and other health risks are at a minimum. In your teens is a little too young. Your body is still growing. The women I talked to in their twenties whose pregnancy was planned definitely seemed less anxious about becoming a mom than older women and less worried about postpartum weight loss—perhaps because career and other life roles had not become established yet. On the other hand, they were less scrupulous about nutrition. Anemia— an iron deficiency—and coping psychologically with an unplanned pregnancy were the greatest problems faced.

Many women today choose not to have children until their thirties. As Kathleen Kelenher says, "The trend today is to postpone child-bearing until the 30s, when women are more likely to have married, settled into a job and come to terms with who they are" ("Through the Ages," *Fit Pregnancy*, Spring 1998, p. 83).

Women in their thirties will probably be less rigid in their approach to becoming a mother and usually have established a life outside of the family. Self-esteem will probably be higher and relationships more stable. On the down side, the risk of delivering babies with birth defects increases as each year passes. After thirty-five the risks go way up. You are more likely to have a C section and deliver prematurely. Also, women in this age range tend to have more anxiety about postpartum weight loss and encounter the biggest problems dealing with it.

Having a baby in your forties carries with it many risks. Medical complications and chromosomal abnormalities increases dramatically. There are benefits, too, though. You may be more comfortable and accepting of your body, more in tune with it. Self-esteem and self-confidence are higher. Women in their forties have a better chance of having healed more of their own childhood wounds, making them much more ready to be present to their own children. "I'd make a much better parent now than before," says Margaret, age 41 and mother of three. You will tend to have a profound respect and wonder for the whole process of creating new life. However, you may also find it harder to lose weight postpartum.

Many first-time mothers are now in their thirties. "These women," writes Paula Siegal in *The Next Nine Months* (Penguin, 1988, p. 188) "will find it harder to lose their excess weight than their twenty-five year old counterparts." Women in their thirties and forties often find pregnancy and new motherhood far more exhausting than younger women. There is less energy for exercise and weight loss. This is especially true if you are breastfeeding. This is because as you age your metabolic rate slows. This means that your body is burning calories at a slower rate than when you were younger.

George Redburn, M.D., an associate professor at Harvard Medical School, told *Redbook* magazine that metabolic rate in women is at its highest around age twenty-seven. After that, it slowly begins to decline. You can't eat what you used to without wearing it on your hips. A declining metabolic rate has nothing to do with childbirth. This would happen anyway. It is just a normal part of aging.

YOUR METABOLIC TYPE

You may not be losing weight postpartum as fast as your friends because your metabolic type is different. How eating and exercise affect your body will be unique to you. When you eat a chocolate bar of 300 calories, it won't have the same caloric effect as on someone else who eats exactly the same chocolate bar. You might put on weight. She might not. Having an awareness of your metabolic rate will help you manage your weight postpartum and what adjustments you need to make in terms of diet and exercise.

Most of us know what our metabolic rate is:

- If you can eat what you want and hardly gain any weight, if you love exercise, and if you find dieting easy, you have a fast metabolic rate.
- If you have to watch what you eat, if you are moderately active, if you lose weight slowly when you diet, you have a moderate metabolic rate.
- If you put on weight very easily, if you find dieting frustrating, if you don't lose weight even when on a diet, and if you don't like exercise, you have a slow metabolic rate.

Hormonal changes in the postpartum period can also affect your metabolic rate. Immediately after pregnancy, your metabolic rate is elevated, but there is also a metabolic change that takes place in the thyroid gland. The adrenal and thyroid glands secrete hormones that influence metabolism. After pregnancy, the thyroid gland reduces hormone production and temporarily slows your metabolism. When this occurs, you will need fewer calories to function.

Your metabolic rate is determined by how much muscle mass you have. Muscles burn calories. After baby, you are more likely to have a higher ratio of fat tissue to muscle tissue than you did before. This higher percentage of fat tissue is going to work against you. If you want to lose weight, you are going to have to start exercising those muscles and increasing your metabolic rate. Exercise is the secret to weight loss postpartum. No amount of dieting will make those pounds disappear if you don't combine it with metabolism-boosting exercise. Remember, though, that you need energy to exercise. Energy is in short supply in the first weeks and months postpartum. Rather than punishing yourself with exercise when you are really too tired, the best thing to do is to use the first few months after baby to rest and regain your strength. Wait until you have your energy back and then start exercising to boost your metabolism.

EMOTIONAL EATING

Do you find yourself turning to food when you are sad, depressed, or angry? If you do, weight loss is going to be tough. Try to keep in mind that you are setting an example for your baby. You want to be a good role model. Now is the time to break the negative chain. You want your child to have a healthy attitude toward food. This has to start with you.

If you feel yourself weakening, be mindful about what you eat. Get away from absolutes. There is no good or bad food. There are only choices. You don't have to make the best food choice, but you can make a good one. If you had too much dessert today, just skip dessert tomorrow. Be good to yourself. Be kind to yourself just as you are to your baby.

THE QUALITY AND QUANTITY OF THE FOOD YOU EAT

If you are having trouble losing weight, try paying close attention to the quality and quantity of the food you are eating. Many of us just have no idea how much we eat and whether or not we are eating nutritiously. Remember the basics of good nutrition you learned while pregnant, and keep a food diary.

Study your diary. See how many of the necessary nutrients you are getting. See how you can start to replace poor nutritional choices with better ones. Compare how much you are eating with the U.S.

Department of Agriculture Food Guide Pyramid (see Figure 7). You might find that you are eating the right foods, but too much of them. Cutting down your serving size will help. Identify what your comfort foods are. If you really can't live without ice cream, be realistic and make a deal to have it not five times but twice a week. You can strike a balance between common sense and indulgence. You don't have to deny yourself; you just have to be sensible.

ERRATIC EATING HABITS

If you have erratic eating habits, you can expect weight loss post-partum to take much longer. Most experts agree that eating smaller, more frequent meals is one of the best ways to adjust to your new appetite and metabolism postpartum

"Skipping meals—especially breakfast—or only eating once a day will not speed up weight loss. It will create metabolic instability and slow down weight loss" (Colleen Sundermeyer, *I Want My Body Back*, Perigee, 1998, p. 24). When you eat food you are using energy through digestion, transportation, and nutrient breakdown. If you fast for long periods, the rate at which you burn calories (your metabolic rate) slows down. It takes far longer to digest the food you do eat. Your body adjusts to eating less food. Thinking your survival is at stake, it will cling onto fat.

If you want to lose weight postpartum, it really does not make sense to go for long periods without food or to go on restrictive diets. Fasting also causes problems with your blood sugar levels, which can trigger mood swings, fatigue, and food cravings.

THE KIND OF PREGNANCY AND DELIVERY YOU HAD

The woman who has had an easy pregnancy and delivery is likely to recover faster than the one who was under strain for nine months.

Was your baby early or late? Was your pregnancy difficult? Were you exhausted all the time? Were there traumatic complications? Was delivery an emotionally and physically exhausting ordeal? Did you have a C section? If you had a C section, your recovery rate will be a little slower initially as your body recovers from the surgery you have had. Most women with C sections have to wait six to eight weeks before they can start easing back into exercise, and even longer before they can begin to do abdominal strengthening exercises.

HOW MANY MONTHS POSTPARTUM YOU ARE

I stopped breastfeeding in the fifth month. My weight stayed the same in the sixth and seventh month, and then in the eighth and ninth month, with no special effort on my part, I lost weight and returned to my prepregnancy weight.

Immediately after delivery and in the first few weeks, your metabolic rate will tend to stay at the higher-than-normal levels of pregnancy. Weight loss is rapid during this time. After a few weeks, though, your metabolic rate settles down to ensure adequate fat storage in case of breastfeeding. That's why weight loss at around two months postpartum, when our bodies are still in baby mode, just doesn't seem to happen.

Between three and six months postpartum, weight loss varies from woman to woman. Some lose, some gain, some stay the same. When weight loss is difficult at a few months postpartum, it is tempting to give up trying to lose weight now. We get despondent. Nothing seems to work. The scales don't change. In frustration, we abandon good eating habits. We put on even more weight. But it is important that you keep eating healthily now. Don't give up. If you just persevere for a few more months, you might start to see results.

Weight loss is easier at about six to nine months postpartum when your metabolic rate has had time to adjust—though it might still be hard for women who are breastfeeding. Leaving weight management later than a year postpartum, though, might be too late.

Studies show that pregnancy pounds that have not been lost a year after giving birth are much less likely to be lost. This excess weight tends to be between five and ten pounds. It is possible to lose it, but it will be much harder to do so. Your body has adjusted to the extra weight.

YOUR MENSTRUAL CYCLE

You will tend not to lose weight until your menstrual cycle becomes regular again. If you still haven't got your periods back, your body is still in a fat storage mode. Fat storage is essential for breastfeeding. Until you start cycling again, your hormones and metabolism are just not at their prepregnancy level. You'll probably find that once you begin to cycle again, weight is easier to lose.

BREASTFEEDING

Your breasts themselves will add a few pounds to the scale. You will hold onto fat stores, too, to ensure milk production. Most women don't return to their prepregnancy weight until they stop breastfeeding. But although you may be a few pounds heavier as long as you nurse, breastfeeding may have long-term benefits for weight management (see next chapter).

YOUR FIRST BABY

Did you enter your pregnancy overweight because you were still recovering from your last baby? Many moms do. The weight isn't lost from the first pregnancy. After each pregnancy, moms tend to gain and keep an average of five to ten pounds.

YOUR LIFESTYLE

How quickly you lose your pregnancy pounds after birth also depends on your lifestyle. Are you working? Are you a stay-at-home mom? One study showed that moms who returned to work outside the home lost weight faster than stay-at-home moms, probably because activity levels increase and food is less readily available. How do you respond to stress? What makes you happy? What makes you sad? What is the best time of day for you? What exercise do you enjoy? What is the food you can't live without? Are you in a relationship? Are you taking oral contraceptives? What star sign are you? Every part of your life will affect how you approach weight management postpartum, and every part needs to be taken into consideration.

How Good a Body Manager Are You?

Let's say you hire a diet and exercise consultant for the first few months postpartum. You tell him your goal is to lose weight. He says you should be able to shape up in six weeks. He does not ask you anything about your life and simply gives you a plan for weight loss. It doesn't work. He says you must be doing something wrong. He says you should have lost the weight—his other clients did. He does not give you a new weight-loss plan. After a few months you are heavier than when before he started. What would you do?

I hope you'd fire him!

But many of us at a few months postpartum are like that terrible fitness manager. We don't take into account how unique we are. We set unrealistic goals. We get despondent. We make comparisons with other moms. We fail to realize that fat stored during pregnancy takes much longer than a few weeks or months postpartum to disappear. In fact, it takes most women about six to nine months postpartum to start seeing weight loss. Nine months on and nine months off is about right.

We need to become better managers of our bodies. Just as you would not put up with poor work from an employee, don't put up with anything less than the best for yourself. Get rid of your old habits and routines, reacquaint yourself with your body, find out what makes you unique. And using the diet and exercise recommendations that follow, design a realistic weight-loss schedule that works for you—and only you.

21

Will I Lose Weight If I Breastfeed?

"Breastfeeding helped me lose weight after the baby."

"I'm nursing and gaining weight. I'm hungry all the time."

"As soon as I stopped nursing, the pounds dropped off."

"I'm losing my postpregnancy weight steadily. I'm still breastfeeding my baby."

You'll get so much conflicting advice. Who do you believe? Does nursing your baby encourage weight loss? Who loses weight the fastest: nursing or bottle-feeding moms?

You have probably talked to moms who swear that breastfeeding helped them lose weight. You will probably have also heard moms say that they couldn't lose weight as long as they breastfed. Who is right?

They both are. Let's look at breastfeeding and bottle-feeding in turn.

Breastfeeding and Weight Loss

"Mothers often wonder if it's possible to lose weight while breastfeeding. The answer is yes. In fact, breast-feeding makes it easier to shed the extra pounds put on in pregnancy. Those pounds were put there after all to store energy for producing milk." This is the pronouncement made by the undisputed "bible" of the breastfeeding movement *The Womanly Art of Breastfeeding* (La Leche League International, Plume, 1997, p. 227).

In the first week postpartum, breastfeeding encourages your uterus to return to its prepregnancy state. You might feel an ache as your uterus contracts when you start nursing. These afterpains are normal. Breastfeeding is speeding up the process of uterine contraction. The benefits for your body don't stop there, though.

Many experts have provided statistics proving that breastfeeding moms lose weight the fastest. Breastfeeding mothers need a lot more calories for the production of milk, so they tend to lose weight without dieting. "Certainly women who breastfeed tend to lose more weight in the first year than those who bottle-feed," write Huggins and Ziedrich in *The Nursing Mother's Guide to Weaning* (Harvard Common Press, 1994, p. 100).

According to Dr. Judith Roepke, a nutritionist in Indiana and a member of the La Leche League Health Advisory Council, nursing is the ideal time to lose weight. If you go into pregnancy a little overweight to start with, nursing may offer you the only opportunity to really get rid of excess weight around the hips and thighs—unless you go for liposuction. It seems that when you are nursing, your body turns to the fat stores in the bottom half of your body for energy to produce milk. Lactation, then, can even mobilize fat that was accumulated before you got pregnant.

Weight loss while breastfeeding must be slow and gradual—otherwise, the quality of milk will be affected adversely. After the first month, safe weight loss is about one or two pounds a month. But if you are patient, eat a sensible, healthy diet, and give your body time to rest, breastfeeding could be one of the best things you have ever done for both you and for baby. Let's look at some of the benefits.

For baby, nursing aids digestion, prevents constipation, lowers the incidence of food allergies, protects baby from infectious diseases, promotes healthy oral development, satisfies suckling needs, and enhances bonding and skin-to-skin contact with mom.

For mom, nursing reduces the chances of hemorrhaging from the placental site, gives mom a chance to rest, encourages the uterus to contract to its prepregnancy size, mobilizes fat for lactation, and enhances bonding and skin-to-skin contact with baby.

Many women swear that the only way for them to lose weight postpartum is to breastfeed. It does make sense. Every time you feed your baby, you are burning up that stubborn fat. You can eat more, too, and not gain weight, as the caloric demands of milk production require more energy.

HOW MANY CALORIES DOES A NURSING MOM NEED?

There is no doubt you should eat more when you are nursing, but how much more is a matter of debate.

It is believed that the average woman between teenage and menopause needs 2,200 calories a day. The current recommendation for mothers who want to breastfeed is 2,700 calories a day if the correct weight was achieved during pregnancy. Those who gained too little need more, and those who gained too much need a little less.

The Food and Nutrition Board, a division of the National Academy of Sciences Institutes, estimates that the average mom makes about 750 milliliters of breast milk a day. It takes around 650 calories to make this milk. Nearly 150 are supposed to come from maternal fat. That means nursing moms need to eat an additional 500 calories a day to maintain their milk supply.

Recent studies, however, have shown that this might be a little too generous. Dr. Nancy Butte, an expert of nutrition and lactation at Children's Research Medical Center at Baylor College of Medicine in Texas, published a ground-breaking study that suggested nursing moms need far less. There are many other factors to take into consideration. Some moms may not produce 750 milliliters of milk a day. Some may not be so efficient at using calories.

There is still uncertainty about how much nursing moms need to eat. The current recommendation ranges from 2,700 to 1,800 calories per day, at the very least. (Note—at 1,800 calories a day, you need to pay extra special attention to getting adequate supplies of the nutrients your baby needs. Never go on a restrictive diet when you are nursing.) The high end of this range may be far too much to let some women lose weight. They may even gain.

It seems that you can lose weight if you aim for around 2,200 calories a day. Although not as generous as a 2,700 calorie allowance, this is definitely a lot more satisfying than the restrictions of some dieting regimes.

NOT ALL NURSING MOMS AUTOMATICALLY LOSE WEIGHT

"I was sure that breastfeeding would help me lose weight. But after five months I was tired, hungry all the time, and gaining rather than losing pounds. I felt like I was a failure."

It would seem that nursing helps weight loss postpartum, but studies show that not all nursing moms automatically lose weight. Even a breastfeeding advocate, Eileen Behan, concludes, "You'll probably lose some weight while you breast-feed, but you may not automatically shed all the weight you put on while you were pregnant" (*Eat Well, Lose Weight While Breastfeeding*, Villard, 1992, p. 68).

The fact is that for some of us, weight loss when breastfeeding is almost impossible. No one is really sure why. It could be that your body chemistry is such that there will be as much fat storage as possible to ensure adequate milk production. Once weaning begins, your biochemistry goes back to normal and it is easier to lose weight. Or, in the words of Dr. Jacobs, "Breastfeeding for weight loss works well in theory. You are using more energy and need more calories. But in practice, it just doesn't work that way. Most women who breastfeed find that they tend to eat more."

LOSING WEIGHT WHEN BREASTFEEDING

Your first priority while breastfeeding is to supply your baby with the nutrients he needs. A poor diet can affect your milk supply. You can't cut down on carbohydrate and fat. Your baby needs the vitamins and minerals they supply. A depletion of your reserves will give you health problems later, too.

If you want to lose weight when you are nursing, you have to resign yourself to the fact that it will be a slow process. You cannot lose weight rapidly. A weight loss of about one to two pounds a month is safe. And this can only be achieved by not eating too much and making the right food choices. Losing weight at this rate may seem painfully slow, but ten months of nursing means ten to fifteen pounds of weight loss. You might find that weight loss plateaus after a few months. This is a common experience and has something to do with how your body stores fat. Weight loss will have to wait until you have weaned. Just make sure you don't start putting on weight.

The good news is that weight that is lost in this gradual, careful way tends to stay off. Study after study has shown that the only really effective way to really lose weight is to lose it gradually and carefully. While you are breastfeeding is the ideal time to start.

Weaning and Weight Loss

A few days after you wean, you will probably lose a few pounds. This will come from your breasts, which probably added a couple of pounds to the scale. You may also find that you aren't constantly hungry all the time and can control your appetite better.

Bottle-feeding and Weight Loss

Bottle-feeding moms and moms who have weaned often find that it is easier to diet and exercise. Your body chemistry returns to normal. You may be able to control your appetite better.

In most cases, bottle-feeding moms can get to their prepregnancy weight faster than breast-feeding moms. The first six weeks are still a time to recover, but after that you can start working on weight loss. Bear in mind, though—your body might need up to six or more months to fully recover from pregnancy, and this may complicate your weight loss plans.

Weight loss is easier because you don't need to be quite so careful about what you do and do not eat. But whether you do lose weight and keep it off is another matter. It depends on your motivation, your diet, your activity levels, and how you lose the weight. Eating sensibly, exercising, and aiming for a gradual weight loss rather than a sudden dramatic one tend to yield the greatest success.

Which Is Best?

In *Bottle-Feeding Without Guilt* (Prima, 1996), Peggy Robin, although never denying that breastfeeding is best, shows that bottle-feeding can be a safe, wise, and beneficial choice if for some reason nursing does not work out. Bonding still occurs. Robin tries to take away the feelings of guilt and inadequacy bottle-feeding moms may experience. She likens the breastfeeding movement to a cult that women feel pressured to join.

As far as weight loss is concerned, an interesting study was conducted by Charles W. Schauberger, M.D., an obstetrician/gynecologist at the Gunderson Clinic in La Crosse, Wisconsin, and his team. Schauberger followed 800 women who breastfed for six months. At six months, only a fifth were still breastfeeding. Schauberger concluded that several factors influenced their weight loss.

- When women went back to work outside the home. At work there is probably less stress, more things to take your mind off food, and less access to food.
- When women get active again. Exercise increases metabolism and works on your fat-to-muscle ratio. The more muscle you have, the more efficiently you will burn calories.
- How old the mother was. Younger moms tend to lose weight faster.
- Oral contraceptives. When women go back on the pill, weight loss can be harder.
- Marital status. Relationships have a big impact on weight management.
- Diet and alcohol consumption.
- Only about 22 percent lost the weight in six weeks, and 37 percent by six months; the remaining 41 percent still carried the excess weight after six months. Schauberger's conclusion: There is no link between weight loss and nursing.

The benefits and disadvantages of breastfeeding and bottle-feeding for baby are outside the scope of this study. (Remember, though, that even manufacturers of formula put on their bottles that "breast is best.") As far as weight loss and breast or bottle-feeding is concerned, the jury is still out. It is clear that the decision to either breastfeed or bottle-feed does affect postpartum weight loss. Weaning from breastfeeding will, too. But this effect will be different for every woman. Once again, it comes down to how individual each woman is. One woman will lose weight quickly while she breastfeeds; another will find her weight stays the same or she even gains a few pounds. Some women who bottle-feed will lose weight fast; others won't. In general, though, if you bottle-feed, you can start losing weight faster than if you breastfeed, when weight loss must be slow and gradual to ensure a nutritious milk supply. Studies have shown, however, that losing weight slowly and gradually is the most successful and effective way to lose weight.

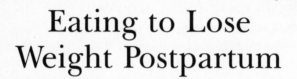

22

Eating to Lose Weight Postpartum

WEIGHT LOSS IS SAFE FOR WOMEN AFTER PREGNANCY AND BREASTFEEDING—but only if diet is balanced and nutritious.

Many diets for weight loss are not nutritionally sound. Restrictive dieting is not a good idea. Not only does it play havoc with your metabolism—depriving the body of food is harmful to the general functioning of your body. Drugs to help you lose weight should be avoided for the same reason and only taken if doctor supervised. Don't get tempted by fad diets that promise miraculous results in a week or two. More often than not, these diets don't give you enough nutrients and do more harm than good.

Studies show that the only really effective way to lose weight is to do it gradually and slowly. You should be aiming for a weight loss of no more than one to two pounds a week or, if breastfeeding, one to two pounds a month.

The First Few Weeks

During the first weeks after giving birth, you will probably be more concerned about your weight than you have ever been. However, you should not even think about dieting until about six weeks. Your body needs adequate nourishment to fully recover from childbirth. Just try to avoid gaining weight. If you are gaining weight, hormonal fluctuations might be the reason, but unhealthy food choices are the more likely cause. A low-fat and low-sugar diet with plenty of fresh fruit, vegetables, whole grains, and lean meat and fish is the wisest food choice you can make now. If you have had a cesarean section, taking vitamin supplements with iron and eating well are especially important now. You have lost a lot more blood than a woman with a vaginal delivery.

Food to Eat During Breastfeeding

A nursing mom needs about 500 additional calories on top of the 2,200 calories believed to be necessary for the average woman of average build. That makes a total of 2,700 calories. If you eat healthily, you will not only be able to feed your baby, but you may also gradually use up the fat supplies you stored during pregnancy for milk production. If you have a lot of excess fat, you can safely restrict your intake to 2,200 calories to lose weight. The lowest safe recommendation for weight reduction is 1,800 calories per day.

It is possible to lose weight when you are breastfeeding, but it is important that this not be done in the first few weeks and that when weight loss occurs, it is slow. Over the first six months, you should lose no more than two pounds a month. This is the amount that won't adversely affect your milk supply. If you lose more, say four or five pounds, your baby won't be getting adequate nutrients, and rapid weight loss may even release toxins stored in your body fat. Never go on a restrictive diet when you are breastfeeding. A nutritious diet is of crucial importance. Good-quality milk is produced from a quality diet and adequate fluid intake.

ESSENTIAL NUTRIENTS DURING BREASTFEEDING

(See Figure 11) Protein is very important for nursing moms, but don't go overboard. About seven ounces of meat, fish, dairy products, and beans and nuts combined with grains is sufficient. Baby needs sufficient protein because it is the basic building block of life from which muscles, skin, bones, and so on are formed.

Vitamin A. Demand for this is high during lactation. Your baby needs it to build a healthy immune system. It also keeps skin healthy. Good food sources are spinach, tomato, apricot, liver, eggs, milk, sweet potato, and carrot. Warning: Vitamin A can be toxic in large amounts.

Vitamin D builds bones for your baby. Good food sources include fish and eggs. Sunlight also helps create vitamin D.

Vitamin E. This is important, especially in the first few months for your baby's muscles and cardiovascular system. Good food sources include nuts, seeds, and green leafy vegetables.

FIGURE 11: ESSENTIAL NUTRIENTS DURING LACTATION

NUTRIENT	RDA PREGNANT	LACTATING RDA, FIRST 6 MONTHS	RDA LACTATING, 6–12 MONTHS
Vitamin A	800 mcg RE	1,300 mcg RE	1,200 mcg RE
Vitamin C	70 mg	95 mg	90 mg
Vitamin D	10 mcg	10 mcg	10 mcg
Vitamin E	10 mg	12 mg	11 mg
Vitamin K	65 mcg	65 mcg	65 mcg
Vitamin B6	2.2 mg	2.1 mg	2.1 mg
Vitamin B12	2.2 mcg	2.6 mcg	2.6 mcg
Thiamine (B1)	1.5 mg	1.6 mg	1.6 mg
Riboflavin (B2)	1.6 mg	1.8 mg	1.7 mg
Niacin (B-3)	17 mg	20 mg	20 mg
Folic Acid	400 mcg	280 mcg	260 mcg
Calcium	1,200 mg	1,200 mg	1,200 mg
Iodine	175 mcg	200 mcg	200 mcg
Iron	30 mg	15 mg	15 mg
Magnesium	320 mg	355 mg	340 mg
Phosphorus	1,200 mg	1,200 mg	1,200 mg
Selenium	65 mcg	75 mcg	75 mcg
Zinc	15 mg	19 mg	16 mg
Protein	60 g	65 g	62 g

RE = retinol equivalents
mg = milligrams
mcg = micrograms

RDA (recommended daily allowance for healthy women) for nutrients increases during breastfeeding

Vitamin K is what makes your baby's blood clot. Your requirement for this won't increase that much during lactation. To eliminate the risk of hemorrhaging after birth, all babies are given a shot of vitamin K. Good sources are green leafy vegetables, milk, meat, eggs, and cereal.

Vitamin C helps your baby fight infection. It can't be stored in your body, so you need to make sure you eat plenty of vitamin C–rich food daily, such as fruits, vegetables, and juice.

Thiamine, vitamin B1, helps you produce breast milk. It is found in beans, nuts, meats, bread, and cereal.

Riboflavin also plays a role in energy production, and it is found in green leafy vegetables, milk, yogurt, and cheese.

Niacin is important for the metabolism of fat and sugar. Good food sources are protein foods, whole-wheat bread, pasta, cereal, and nuts.

Vitamin B6. This is vital for you and baby. It assists in the metabolism of protein and fat and in the production of red blood cells. Good sources of vitamin B6 include bananas, potatoes, cauliflower, soybeans, and shellfish.

Folic acid helps form red blood cells and build new ones. It is essential during pregnancy. During lactation, your requirement drops, but eating folic acid foods is still important. Food sources include green leafy vegetables, beans, seeds, eggs, and wheat germ.

Vitamin B12 works with folic acid to create healthy red blood cells. You can meet your vitamin B12 requirements by eating animal foods, soy milk, and B12-fortified cereal.

Calcium is essential for strong bones and teeth. Your body will ensure that your baby gets enough calcium, but if your calcium intake is low, it will do this at your expense. Your body will release calcium from your bones to make up the difference. Most calcium-rich foods are dairy products, but other sources are broccoli, fish, and tofu.

Phosphorus. This is needed for adequate calcium absorption. What you eat won't affect your phosphorus level much, but good food sources are animal foods and soft drinks.

Magnesium helps with the release of energy and helps with proper muscle function. Good sources are green vegetables, nuts, seeds, legumes, and whole grains.

Iron is important for the circulation of oxygen in the blood. You need less than when you were pregnant, but you still need it, especially if your periods have started. Good sources are spinach, eggs, beans, shellfish, liver, and red meat.

Zinc. Your needs for this are very high in the first few months of lactation. Zinc helps maintain the health of many organs in the body. As with calcium, if your breast milk is deficient, your body will drain zinc from your stores. You can find zinc in poultry, seafood, whole grains, and black-eyed peas.

Iodine for thyroid function. Your thyroid regulates body temperature and metabolism. Iodine is in seafood and plant-fed animals. Your requirements for iodine increase during lactation.

Selenium works with vitamin E. You do need more than if you were not breastfeeding. It is found in seafood and grains.

Fluid. Inadequate fluid intake is associated with a reduction in milk supply. Making sure you drink enough water is important.

Supplements

Nutrient requirements do increase during lactation. For example, daily requirements for vitamin A and vitamin C nearly double when you are nursing. The same applies to zinc and iodine. On the other hand, requirements for folic acid fall to just above your prepregnancy amounts. If you are eating a well-balanced diet, most of the nutrients should be readily available, but doctors often recommend that you take vitamin and mineral supplements, especially for the first six months when baby's demand for nutrients is at its highest.

- Calcium, zinc, magnesium, vitamin B6, and folic acid are the nutrients that nursing moms are most likely to be deficient in.
- If diet is restricted or low-calorie, deficiencies are likely in calcium, zinc, magnesium, vitamin B6, folic acid, thiamine, iron, vitamin E, riboflavin, selenium, and niacin.
- Vitamin A, vitamin B6, vitamin D, iodine, and selenium can be harmful if overconsumed.

Weight Loss After Breastfeeding

If you didn't breastfeed or have stopped breastfeeding, you don't have to worry anymore that the food you eat will affect your baby's health. All moms, though, should continue to eat a healthy, balanced diet with all the essential nutrients.

Having excess weight can be avoided by eating a diet that keeps you in the range of a weight that is desirable for you. Excess weight results from an imbalance between energy intake and energy expenditure. Effective weight loss occurs when you eat fewer calories to burn up fat stores and increase your activity levels. "These two elements are the cornerstones of natural, self directed, weight loss regimes" (Stavia Blunt, *Shaping up During and after Pregnancy*, Summersdale, 1997, p. 51).

CALORIE REDUCTION

Many moms want to know how many calories a day they should be eating for weight loss. The average woman is supposed to use up around 2,200 calories a day. So if calories were restricted by 500 a day, a weight loss of between 0.5 and 2 pounds a week can be expected, depending, of course, on activity levels. No woman should consume less than 1,200 calories a day. If you underfeed your body, it will start to store calories as fat, and if you eat less than 1,200 calories, you probably won't be getting the nutrients your body needs to stay healthy.

Rather than focusing on calories, though, weight loss tends to be more effective when the focus is on nutrition. Pregnancy has shown you that your body knows what to do. That you can trust it. That sensible eating can yield wonderful results. This does not mean throwing caution to the wind and eating all you want; it means trusting your instincts more. Paying attention to how you feel when you eat and to what is best for your body, not to how many calories you are eating. True, a reduction in the amount of calories you eat will help you lose weight. But too much focus on calories can be a frustrating experience. No two calories are the same. The calories you get in a banana are very different from the calories you get from a handful of sweets. Both might have the same number of calories, but the banana has more nutrient value. You need nutrients to stay healthy and energized.

A Nutritionally Sound Postpartum Food Plan

It is important that new moms consume all the essential nutrients (see Chapter Six). I advise against it, but if you must count calories and want to lose weight, make sure that your calorie count consists of 20 to 30 percent protein, 40 to 60 percent carbohydrate, and 20 to 30 percent fat.

You need a balance of all the essential nutrients (proteins, carbo-hydrates, fats, water, vitamins, minerals) to feel healthy and to lose weight effectively. Let's look at this in more detail.

Although protein is not quite as vital as during pregnancy, if you don't get enough in your postpartum diet, your body will break down its own muscle tissue, and the result will be loss of muscle tone, thinning hair, food cravings, and fatigue. Proteins are also important for weight loss because they stimulate glucagon, which restores blood sugar levels and releases fat. Protein increases metabolic rate, helps burn fat, and gives you energy. Protein is found in foods like lean meat, fish, eggs, milk, beans, nuts, yeast, grains, soy, and wheat germ. But getting too much protein is not advisable, either. You might have heard a lot about high-protein, low-carbohydrate diets. While it is true that increased amounts of protein will stimulate metabolic rate and help you burn fat, these diets don't tend to be effective. When you cut down on carbohydrates, your body turns to muscles for fuel. You lose muscle mass, and you'll be using fewer calories.

In recent years, the emphasis has been on high-carbohydrate and low-fat diets. The standard recommendation was to make carbohydrate 70 percent of your diet. The trouble with this is that carbohydrate not converted immediately by the body into sugar and used is stored as fat. You will still put on weight. The kinds and amounts of carbohydrate eaten are very important if you are trying to lose weight. Starch is a good source of carbohydrate and it is found in bread, potatoes, rice, pasta, fruit, vegetables, and cereal. Sucrose (table sugar) is not a good source of carbohydrate, but the natural sugars found in fruit and veg-etables are. Good sources of carbohydrate are often high in fiber, which is essential for effective weight loss, as it plays an important part in reg-ular bowel movements. Good sources of fiber are whole-grain bread, pasta, vegetables, and fruit. Opinions differ but many nutritionists think that starch and fiber should be about 40 to 50 percent of your diet, especially if you are trying to lose weight.

Low-fat diets and low-sugar diets are also very popular, probably because our fat and sugar consumption is way too high. But cutting down on them too much is not good, either. Fats keep the body func-tioning and you need a certain amount of fat to burn fat. Saturated fats are mainly of animal origin. They are found in meat, milk, butter and cheese, and nuts. They should be taken in moderation, as they can raise blood cholesterol to dangerous levels. Polyunsaturated and monounsaturated fats have greater health benefits. They tend to occur in plants and soy oil, and they lower blood cholesterol. Fish and seaweed, flaxseed oil, green leafy vegetables, liver, and olive oil are other good sources.

It is also important to ensure an adequate intake of water. Our bodies are about two-thirds water, so the intake and distribution of fluid is important for weight loss. If the body is deprived of water, blood volume is reduced and does not circulate to the tissues as effectively. The brain is most affected, and you might feel dizzy. You will almost certainly feel fatigued if you are dehydrated. The solution is to drink enough water. Six to eight glasses a day is recommended.

Reducing or eliminating the amount of caffeine and alcohol is also important if weight loss is your goal. Alcohol can cause high blood pressure, and caffeine and cigarettes, although they temporarily boost metabolism, can cause stress, fatigue, headaches, and lack of energy. Caffeine and alcohol also deplete the body of water and minerals because they have a diuretic effect and hinder the efficient metabolism of food.

If you eat a balanced, healthy, diet with proper attention to serving size (see later), you will almost certainly lose weight. However, many moms who go on diets often find it hard to get all the vitamins and minerals they need for the normal functioning of their bodies and for effective weight loss. Make sure your diet includes an adequate vitamin and mineral intake. If it doesn't, a supplement is wise.

Figure 12 gives a list of Recommended Dietary Allowances adapted from the Food and Nutrition Board of the National Academy of Sciences. The RDAs, however, are surprisingly controversial, and you will often see suggested RDAs differ from expert to expert. As things stand now, the RDAs prevent most nutrient deficiency diseases, but many scientists believe they should be substantially increased to reflect the mounting evidence that larger doses of vitamins and minerals can prevent and treat many diseases.

The RDAs are about to be replaced by new guidelines, the Dietary Reference Intakes (DRI), issued by the Food and Nutrition Board (FNB) that determines the RDAs. Two RDAs have already been dramatically increased—calcium and folic acid. It is still not OK, though, to take large doses of vitamin and mineral supplements. (See Chapter Seven.)

FIGURE 12: RDA VITAMIN AND MINERAL REQUIREMENTS

NUTRIENT	RDA (RECOMMENDED DAILY ALLOWANCE)
Vitamin A	800 mcg RE
Vitamin B1	1.1 mg
Vitamin B2	1.3 mg
Vitamin B3	15 mg
Vitamin B6	1.6 mg
Vitamin B12	2.0 mcg
Folic acid	180 mcg
Vitamin C	50 mg
Vitamin D	5 mcg
Vitamin E	8 mg
Vitamin K	65 mcg
Calcium	800 mg
Iodine	150 mcg
Iron	15 mg
Magnesium	280 mg
Phosphorus	800 mg
Selenium	55 mcg
Zinc	12 mg
Protein	50 g

RE = retinol equivalents
mg = milligrams
mcg = micrograms

SERVING SIZE

Proper attention paid to serving size will encourage the slow, gradual weight loss you should aim for. Start checking your servings now and make a few small reductions in what you're eating. Even the smallest reductions will help you lose weight. You don't need to cut out your favorite dishes or sweets—just don't eat too much of them, because eating too much is the most likely cause of weight gain. If you're trying to slim down, watch your portion sizes. For the grain group, for instance, every slice of bread or half-cup of rice counts for one serving. The large bowl of spaghetti you had last week might have had as many as seven servings. The standard portion size in America has gotten bigger and bigger. As a result, waistlines have gotten bigger, too.

If you follow the USDA food guide pyramid for serving size (Figure 7), you should be getting a balanced diet with sufficient vitamins and minerals. It won't be on the bestseller list, but the U.S. Department of Agriculture's food guide pyramid is still the best guideline for a healthy diet.

Fats, oils and sugar. You don't need to cut these out entirely, but you do need to eat them in moderation. It is fine to enjoy chocolate doughnuts once in a while. It is not fine to enjoy them every day.

Breads, cereals, rice, and pasta. One serving is one slice of bread, one ounce of cereal, or half a cup of rice or pasta. The grain group supplies you with carbohydrates for energy, vitamins and minerals, and fiber. The recommendation is between 6 and 11 servings a day of bread, rice, pasta, or cereal. If you are trying to lose weight, 6 or 7 servings might be right. High-fiber foods, such as brown rice and whole-grain breads and cereals, are important in this group because they fill up and regulate your digestive system.

Vegetables. Aim for at least two nutrient-rich servings, preferably more. One serving is half a cup of raw or cooked vegetables.

Fruit. Aim for about four nutrient-rich servings, preferably more. One serving is one piece of fruit.

Milk, yogurt and cheese. Two or three servings should be sufficient. One serving is about two ounces of cheese or one cup of milk or yogurt.

Meat, fish, beans, eggs, nuts. Two or three servings should be sufficient. One serving is about three ounces of meat or fish, one egg, or half a cup of beans.

Avoiding large meals and changing your routine to smaller, more frequent snacks will also help now. Around six small meals a day is about right. Why is this beneficial for weight loss? Because overeating at any one time overloads your system with sugar and fat. Fasting for too long between meals slows your metabolism. Most nutritionists agree that eating little and often is one of the most effective ways to promote weight loss.

Nutrient-Rich Foods

If you want to lose weight postpartum, cut down on foods that have little nutritional value and consume more nutrient-rich foods. Foods rich in nutrients have magic properties that can eliminate hunger, erase water weight, and speed up your body's fat-burning power. The more nutrient-rich foods you eat, the slimmer you will get. You won't feel hungry all the time either. Here are a few examples of nutrient-rich foods that can actually help you lose weight.

- Whole grain bread. This has chromium, the metabolism-boosting mineral that helps you shed stored fat. It also contains iron, which plays an important part in the burning of energy from the food you eat.
- Whole wheat bread. This contains niacin, which helps release the energy from the food you eat.
- Bananas. Bananas contain potassium. Potassium flushes sodium out of the body and can help you lose weight. Women who have more potassium in their diet burn calories faster than those who don't. Bananas and cantaloupe are good food sources. Bananas also contain magnesium, which is indispensable for weight loss. It is involved in every major biological process in the body.
- Sweet potatoes. These contain complex carbohydrates, which create fat burning muscle. They also have vitamin A, which is important for carbohydrate metabolism.
- Broccoli. Broccoli and carrots are low in calories. Your body burns calories simply by chewing them. Broccoli also contains vitamins B2 and B6, which are essential for carbohydrate and fat metabolism and the breakdown of protein.
- Black-eyed peas. High in zinc. Zinc is an important nutrient for weight loss. It is associated with the functioning of insulin, the hormone that regulates carbohydrate metabolism.
- Spinach. Contains iodine, which is important for weight loss and helps the body metabolize excess fat.
- Lean meats. The protein in lean meat such as chicken helps you convert fat into muscle. Muscle burns more calories than fat. Protein also takes longer to digest than carbohydrate, so eating it keeps you satisfied longer and prevents snacking.
- Water. Drink lots of water when trying to lose weight. Increasing your water intake can help flush out water weight. Cold water also uses up a lot of calories when your body tries to warm it, but some doctors recommend not shocking the body that way.
- Fiber-rich foods. Foods like kidney beans, fiber-rich vegetables, and bran cereals expand in our stomachs, filling us up with fewer calories. Adequate fiber ensures healthy digestion. It can block the absorption of fat, too.
- Eggs. Rich in biotin, which is needed for the release of energy from carbohydrates, for fat burning, and for the breakdown of amino acids. Biotin is essential for weight loss. (Other food sources of biotin include legumes, milk, cereal, and nuts.) Eggs

also contain vitamin B5, which is important for energy and tissue metabolism. Eggs have phosphorus, too, which is needed for the normal function of many of the B vitamins involved in energy production. The whites of eggs are protein sources that contain the amino acid L-carnitine, which studies have shown unlocks the fat stored in our cells and enables it to be burned for energy.

- Strawberries. Like all fruits, strawberry is high in vitamin C. Vitamin C is essential for weight loss. It is involved in the metabolism of amino acids.
- Whole-wheat pasta. This boosts serotonin levels. Serotonin is the feel-good hormone that can stop food cravings.
- Green leafy vegetables. These are high in vitamin E. If you want to lose weight, you must eat foods rich in vitamin E. Vitamin E protects your body from toxins when you lose weight.

Foods to Avoid

Avoid foods that make you feel bloated. Synthetic food additives, processed foods, foods high in salt, coffee, and chocolate will make you feel bloated and heavy.

If you feel bloated a lot of the time, start eating more good-quality, wholesome foods that are free of additives and rich in nutrients. Don't fill your shopping cart with fast food that is refined, processed, and packed with sodium and synthetic additives. These kinds of food just don't have the necessary vitamins and minerals you need for weight loss. Instead, concentrate on whole, unrefined, and fresh foods that are rich in nutrients.

Change Your Eating Habits for Life

In order to lose weight postpartum, most of us will have to change our eating habits. More fruit and vegetables, less fat and sugar, reduction in serving size, and an adequate intake of the nutrients you need are the best and most effective ways to lose weight.

Time and time again, when women go on diets, weight is lost and then gained back again. If you want to lose your baby fat and keep it off, it is vital that you don't go back to your old eating patterns. If you do, the weight will pile back on again. Instead of thinking about dieting after baby, think more in terms of a permanent change in eating habits. From now on, you are going to eat to maximize your chances not just of permanent weight loss, but of good health and vitality, too.

23

Exercise for Postpartum Weight Loss

"Exercise helped me lose weight. I was back to my prepregnancy weight in three months."

"Exercise was vital for me in the post partum recovery period."

"Without a regular exercise program, I know I would not have lost the weight."

"Getting active again made me feel better about myself."

You might think that having a child would increase your activity levels, but recent studies show that the reverse is true. Moms tend to exercise less. But if you want to lose weight postpartum, exercise, in combination with a balanced diet, is key. You can lose weight by diet alone, but without exercise, you might still look flabby and out of shape. Exercise gives you tone and shape. It helps your stomach and waist tighten up and makes your hips look firmer. Lack of muscle tone in the abdominals and pelvic area leave you at risk of backache and stress incontinence. In the past it was thought that this was an unavoidable part of childbearing. We know better today. We know that exercise can correct muscle weakness caused by pregnancy and if not prevent, at least improve various related disorders.

Exercise itself burns calories, but what is more important is that you build up muscle mass through exercise. Muscles burn calories more efficiently than fat. The more lean muscle tissue you have, the higher your metabolism will be. The higher your metabolism, the faster you will lose weight and burn up fat stores. After pregnancy most moms have more fat stored than at any other time in their lives. Most of this will disappear naturally in the postpartum months, but those last stubborn pounds can often only be lost through increasing activity levels.

Exercise encourages body awareness. You will be more in tune with the many changes going on in your body in the postpartum period. There are other benefits, too. Exercise improves cholesterol profile and decreases the risk of diabetes, heart disease, and breast and colon cancer. It eases the discomforts of PMS and helps fight colds and infections better. It can reduce back pain. It helps build bones and calorie-burning muscles, thus promoting weight loss. It may even make you feel sexier and live longer. It also "improves strength, sleeping patterns and self-esteem," says Donna Meltzer, M.D., a clinical assistant professor in the Department of Family Medicine at State University of New York at Stony Brook (quoted from *Fit Pregnancy*, Spring 1999, p. 103).

Exercise is, in fact, the best thing you can do for yourself in the postpartum period. As well as helping you lose weight and regain muscle tone, especially in the abdominal and pelvic region, exercise has emotional benefits. It can help you build self-esteem and improve your body image.

A Gentle Start

In the first six weeks, you probably won't have the time or the energy for exercise. You will want to rest as much as you can. Don't worry. Rest is important—it will help you recover faster. Take every opportunity to rest when you can. Wait until you feel a little stronger and until your doctor says you can exercise. Enjoy your baby. These precious moments soon pass.

Although lots of activity in the first few months postpartum is not recommended, gentle exercise is, because it can speed your recovery. Biking and running are out. Your muscles and connective tissue need to heal and to regain strength, and your joints are vulnerable to injury. All you should think about right now are your abdominal muscles, your pelvic muscles, and your back muscles, and correcting your posture.

Whatever kind of labor you had, you can probably begin some simple exercises in the first few days:

1. Kegels. Contract the muscles around your vagina and hold for 10 seconds. If you are not sure what you should be feeling, the next time you urinate hold the flow for a few moments. Aim for five or so sets of ten repetitions, a couple of times a day. Kegels will help you strengthen your pelvic floor muscles. The great thing about them is that you can do them anytime, anywhere.

2. Easy abdominals. Lie on your back and bend your knees with your feet on the floor. Take a deep breath and as you exhale, tighten your abdominal muscles and hold the contraction for about five seconds. Do about ten or twenty of these a day to strengthen your abdominals.

3. Pelvic tilt. Lie on your floor with knees bent and feet flat on the floor. Keep knees and feet together and gently tighten the muscles in your buttocks. Roll your pelvis up and hold for a moment. Tighten your abdominals as you perform the pelvic tilt and push your back into the floor. Repeat twenty times. This really helps ease backache and is great for posture.

4. Wall sit. Lean against a wall and slide down so you are in a sitting position. Try to sit for ten seconds and build up slowly to thirty seconds. This will strengthen your thighs.

5. Stretching. On all fours with knees under hips, arms under shoulders, and back straight, round your spine, tucking your tailbone underneath you and relaxing your head and neck to stretch your back. Return to neutral, slightly arching spine, with head up. This will stretch and strengthen your back.

6. Posture. Hold your back straight and your head high. Proper posture will prevent you straining your back when your abdominal muscles and back muscles are weak. This is especially important as you place a lot of strain on your back in the early months with bending and lifting your baby.

7. Try to walk for at least five minutes in the first few days. This will help you recover faster.

Provided you had no complications during labor and had a relatively straightforward vaginal delivery, you can start walking and doing simple tasks again. Get out and walk as much as you can and take your baby with you. Stop and rest at the first sign of tiredness.

At about two weeks you can start a very easy exercise program, but make sure it *is* easy and that you warm up, cool down, and stretch properly. If you are nursing, drink a lot of fluids. Avoid any high-impact exercise, such as jogging, and exercises such as cycling if you had an episiotomy. Stop if you feel any pain. Stop if you feel any tiredness. You can walk, or do low-intensity exercises like stair climbing or riding a stationary bike. All these exercises are low impact. You can modify them to suit how you are feeling. You probably won't want to start swimming again until your bleeding stops, because doctors advise that you use pads and not tampons for postpartum bleeding.

You may be eager to do much more, but there are reasons why intense exercise can wait a couple of weeks until your body is ready. It is not until at least six weeks postpartum that your uterus returns to its normal size. Exercising too soon increases the risk of prolapse of the uterus. The muscles that supported your uterus during pregnancy, called the pelvic floor muscles, also need to heal, and if you plan to nurse, you need time to establish a nursing routine. Ligaments and joints are vulnerable. Although bleeding is normal in the first few weeks, you will know if you are doing too much exercise if bleeding is heavy and continues for longer than four weeks postpartum.

If you were very fit and active before and during your pregnancy, you might be able to resume an active program before your six-week checkup. But you need to listen to your body, talk to your doctor, and start your exercise program gradually. Your aim is to get fit and healthy again, not to get injured and exhausted. Don't be tempted to do too much too soon. "It takes a good four to six weeks for the hormones of pregnancy to get out of your system," says Dr. Jacobs. "If you start working out too soon, your body is just not ready, and you risk prolapse of the uterus and other complications. Walking is fine the day after delivery. Non-weight-bearing exercise is fine. But it is vital that you start gradually to let your body adjust, and don't do anything vigorous in these early weeks."

At Six Weeks

At six weeks, provided your doctor is happy with your progress, getting back to an exercise routine is safe. That is, assuming you have the energy to start one. You probably won't be up to a forty-five minute aerobic class yet. Don't get frustrated. Remember, you have just had a baby. Give your body time to heal and to get strong again. Most moms I talked to just did not have the energy for exercise in the early months. And those who did, said that they exercised at a less intense level than before they were pregnant. A good postnatal exercise class might be a good idea. These classes are designed to work on postpregnancy weaknesses and build up your strength gradually so that you can get back to your prepregnancy fitness levels.

The keys to successful recovery to your prepregnancy fitness levels are to take things slowly and listen to your body. For example, you can start walking briskly with light weights before you jog or do aerobics. Start with twenty minutes and build up to an hour. Let how you feel be the guide. You will know when you are ready to include more jarring activities, such as running, into your exercise program.

How long it takes to feel fit again is very individual. Some women can get fit again in a matter of months, but most of us take about a year. Some women say that they never got their fitness levels back, but others say that their fitness improved. I even read about many Olympic runners who improved their time one to two years after having a baby. Pregnancy brought focus to their training.

Postpartum Exercise Programs

Provided you have no physical problems and you can find the time, energy, motivation, and discipline to exercise regularly, there is no reason why you shouldn't get back to your prepregnancy fitness levels. For weight loss, increased energy, physical strength, and an overall feeling of well-being, exercise postpartum is a must.

You may not have the time or the inclination to join a gym, so here's some advice about how you can design an effective weight management exercise program yourself. Your program should include aerobic activity, muscle strengthening, and stretching.

AEROBIC EXERCISE

Lack of regular aerobic exercise is the main cause of weight gain. Aerobic exercise means exercising with oxygen repeatedly for an extended period of time so that your body starts burning fat. You should be slightly out of breath, but not so much that you can't carry on a conversation when you exercise aerobically. If you exercise too hard, you won't lose weight. Muscle size will increase too much, and water weight will be retained. Aerobic exercises include brisk walking, jogging, swimming, cycling, skiing, rowing, stair climbing, roller skating, aerobic dance classes, step classes, and boxing. A 150-pound individual can burn around 500 to 750 calories an hour doing aerobic exercise of moderate intensity such as fast walking, jogging, swimming, aerobic dance, and cycling; 250 to 500 calories an hour for aerobic activity of lower intensity such as walking at a slow pace or golf; and 750 to 900 calories an hour with higher intensity exercise such as vigorous sports—squash or rope jumping, for example. If you weigh less you'll burn slightly less, and if you weigh more you'll burn more.

After pregnancy you have to start burning up the excess fat that your body has stored. To do this you have to exercise aerobically several times a week. Keep going for more than twenty minutes and no more than an hour. There seems to be something magic about the twenty-minute mark. After about twenty minutes, your body switches from burning mainly carbohydrate for energy to burning mainly fat for energy. That's why programs that recommend you exercise for twenty minutes three times a week are rarely able to help you lose weight. Twenty minutes might be enough to improve the condition of your heart and lungs, but it's not enough time to burn extra fat.

Start with twenty minutes of aerobic exercise and build up to forty-five minutes or an hour three to five times a week. Fit in your aerobic exercise whenever you can. Many moms get up very early so that they can have this time to exercise. You might be able to exercise while your baby is napping, or you could get a sitter. Whatever it takes, any new mom who is serious about weight management needs to make exercise a part of her life.

STRENGTH TRAINING

To burn fat, you need to get your strength back, too, and build up your muscles. Muscles need more energy than fat. As well as helping you manage your weight, strength training helps fight the effects of aging (we lose muscle strength as we age), gives you more energy, and gives your body shape and tone. Training for strength means working your muscles harder than they normally do with lifting, pulling, and pushing. Most gyms would be able to help you with a strength training program with weights or machines, but there are many alternatives that achieve the same results—yoga, pilates (an exercise technique), or calisthenics for example. Or you may choose to do exercises on your own.

You can work on your abdominals with slow and careful abdominal crunches. Lie on your back with knees bent, lift your head and shoulders up, and then return them to the floor. Oblique abdominals where you twist at your waist to reach the opposite knee, as well as abdominal curls where you lie on your back with your knees in the air and gently raise your hips off the floor and down again, will also help strengthen and tone your stomach muscles. Making a habit of tightening your abdominal muscles whenever you can and holding for a few seconds can also be effective. To get the best results from abdominal exercises, do them slowly. That way your muscles have to work harder. If you do them quickly, other muscles in your legs and upper body end up working out, and your abs don't get a workout. Remember, though—if you want those firm abs to be seen, you have to burn off the excess flab hiding them with aerobic exercise.

To trim the thighs, slide down a wall with your back straight until you reach a sitting position and hold for about thirty seconds. Squats will strengthen your buttocks, hamstrings, and quadriceps. Buttock clenches where you squeeze your buttock muscles for a few seconds will help tone those buttocks, too. Kegels help the pelvic floor area, and press-ups, where you kneel down on all fours and bend and straighten your arms, will build up your pectoral muscles and make your breasts look firmer.

Make sure that before you do any strength training exercises, you warm up and stretch for about ten minutes beforehand and cool down and stretch afterwards.

STRETCHING

After having a baby you may feel more flexible than you have ever been. It's still important to keep stretching though. As we get older we get stiffer and our muscles are not so elastic anymore. Stretching reduces the chance of injury and encourages ease of movement. If your aim is to have a long, lean dancer-like body, stretching and lengthening your body is vital.

Calf stretching where you feel the stretch in your calf by leaning against a wall, or pressing your heels down on a step, is important to do before aerobic exercise. Lying on your back and drawing your knees into your chest will stretch the lower back. There are also stretches for the front and back of your thighs, your hips, chest, shoulders, and arms. One of the easiest and most beneficial stretches is a whole body stretch. Put your hands in the air, rise up onto your toes, and stretch as hard as you can as if you were trying to reach something.

NO TIME TO EXERCISE

"I don't have time." This is the complaint I hear most often from new moms. But there are ways you can find the time. You could think about a babysitter, or find a gym that has child-care facilities. You could try to fit in exercise when you can. Even a few minutes of exercise a few times a day is beneficial. Try to exercise when baby naps (if he does nap!) or work out with baby watching. Try placing your baby in a swing, car seat, or stroller or exerciser when you exercise. (For every five attempts at exercise, he might be content to watch you for at least one of them.) Many moms also get up before baby to fit their exercise in. There are exercise videos to choose from. My advice is to buy three or four and alternate them. It's easy to get bored with the same class and routine. You could also try mother and baby exercise routines. Some moms say this works for them. Try, if you can, to get your baby involved. Take him for walks in the stroller. Carry him in a back pack. Play with him between stretching and strengthening exercises. Talk to him when you are doing them.

AND FOR THOSE WHO HATE EXERCISE

If joining a gym does not appeal to you, if you hate the idea of an exercise program you must stick to, there is salvation. You can incorporate toning and strengthening exercise to build muscle mass into your daily life—for example, tightening your buttocks when you can or pulling in your tummy and working on your posture. Putting more energy into everyday chores such as housework can also burn calories and tone muscles. Make your daily life a little more active, and don't sit around too much watching your baby. You might like to try walking more.

WALKING

Walking doesn't really seem like exercise, but the benefits of regular walking are incredible. It's one of the best forms of exercise for new moms. You can take your baby along. You can walk indoors or outdoors if the weather isn't good. Baby will enjoy the fresh air and scenery change. You can start walking within days after delivery, but wait until your six-week checkup before you get really serious. Walking also tones your stomach and bottom. Best of all, walking burns calories. If you walk a mile or two every day at a brisk pace, you can lose a couple of pounds a month, especially if this is combined with a sensible diet.

If you start walking regularly with a stroller as a way of losing weight, try to walk at a pace that makes your heart beat just a little faster, but not too much. For fat burning, you should aim to walk at least five times a week. It won't harm you to walk every day as long as you don't push yourself too hard. The question of how often is less important than how long you walk.

When you start a walking plan, try walking for ten minutes a few times a day. Keep an easy pace and let your body tell you how you feel. If you can go a little faster, try it. You're going too fast if you can't carry a conversation without gasping. Slow down if you need to. The aim is to build up your endurance so that in a year's time you will be walking briskly for forty minutes or more. Try to keep your back straight and your abdominal muscles contracted with your tailbone down. Cool down by reducing your pace again, and then finish with stretches that you hold for about thirty seconds without bouncing.

If your schedule is tight and long walks seem impossible, recent research is suggesting that several short walks may help you lose weight because it may boost your calorie burn throughout the day. But most fitness experts still believe that longer walks are more effective for weight loss and for endurance and increased fitness.

A Word on Posture

What's the quickest way to look taller, thinner, and healthier postpartum?

Simple: practice good posture. If you are feeling fat, poor posture can make you feel even worse. Poor posture can make even thin people look flabby. Keeping the body aligned from head to toe is more than a matter of mere vanity. It also substantially reduces the risk of pain and injury, especially in the lower back. New moms spend most of the day bending, lifting, and carrying. All this places great strain on your back.

You may have gotten into bad habits during pregnancy when the weight of your baby pushed your center of gravity forward. Bad habits can be hard to break. You'll probably make the problem worse when your baby is old enough to be carried on your hip. The curve in your lower back gets worse. The pressure on your spine intensifies.

To check your posture, have a look at yourself sideways in a mirror. Pull your shoulders back, tuck your buttocks under, lift your head and chin up, and feel as if someone is pulling you from the center of your head with a string. If you really take the time to do this exercise, you'll realize how used to being slumped you are. You'll also see how good posture can take pounds off you and make you look more confident and poised. It's an old trick, but walking for a few minutes a day with a book on your head can really help you pull up and stand tall.

Perfect posture is not easy, and you won't be able to think of it all the time, but you really are doing yourself a service every time you do a posture check and readjust how you are sitting, standing, or bending. Working on your posture is a strengthening exercise all in itself. You will be surprised—the more you pull up and stand tall with your weight balanced correctly, the trimmer and firmer you will look. Good posture is crucial to your well-being. Life with chronic back pain is not pleasant. Make sure you buy a stroller that is the right height for you, one that you don't have to bend to push. When you bend to lift your baby, bend at the knees and try not to carry your baby on your hip too much.

Exercise and Breastfeeding

It is important if you do exercise and breastfeed that you eat enough to supply the demands of exercise and enough to produce an adequate milk supply. It might be hard to find the time in the first six weeks, when you are establishing your milk supply, to begin regular exercise that won't compromise the time you need for nursing.

As long as you exercise moderately and eat enough calories, your breast milk will not be affected. "Breastfeeding and exercise are compatible. There is no evidence that exercise will diminish the quality of your milk," writes Joan Marie Butler in *Fit and Pregnant* (Acorn, 1996, p. 161). Sensible exercise won't affect your milk supply. You might find it challenging to run with leaking, tender, and larger breasts, but it should not stop you from exercising moderately. Make sure you invest in a good sports bra. Cotton is better than synthetic fabrics, which can cause irritation. Buy a bra with lots of support and strong straps.

The best time to exercise is immediately after you have breastfed your baby. Some studies have concluded that changes in the composition of the milk might occur right after exercising. Other studies contradict this and even show that breastfeeding moms who exercise have a higher milk volume than nonexercising moms. "After reviewing many studies of breastfeeding mothers who exercise, researchers concluded that moderate exercise during breastfeeding is safe and beneficial for most women" (*The Womanly Art of Breastfeeding*, Plume, 1997, p. 227).

Exercise and C Sections

Most doctors advise waiting till your first postoperative checkup—which is about two weeks after an uncomplicated C section—before attempting any exercise. Lifting anything heavier than your baby is also not recommended. However, they will encourage light exercise as soon as the evening after a morning surgery.

You'll spend the first few days in the hospital learning how to shift your body without using your abdominal muscles. This will take some time, so don't get depressed if it takes quite a few attempts. Your nurses will encourage you to stand up straight even if you feel pain. They are not being unsympathetic. They know that crouching over won't help you heal—it restricts your blood supply and makes healing take longer. In the early days, a binder might help you, but you shouldn't start to rely on it. You need to get your abdominal strength back as soon as possible.

Rest is important in the first few days to speed recovery, but you also need to start some kind of gentle exercise, even though it might be painful at first. Walking improves circulation in your legs and stops blood clots forming. It also gets bowel function back, allowing gas to work its way down. Kegels will begin getting your pelvic floor muscles back into shape. You can do these almost immediately after surgery. Other gentle exercises you can do include the following:

- Leg slides to help support your abdominals. Lie on your back with legs extended, slide one foot up toward your buttocks, and bend your knee. Press the small of your back into the floor and slide the leg out again. Then slide the other leg up toward the buttocks and do the same.
- The pelvic tilt. Bend your legs at the knees with your feet flat on the bed. Gently roll your lower spine up, clench your buttocks, and then roll down again until your back is flat again.
- Belly breathing. During surgery your respiratory tract may start to collect excess mucus and fluid. For that reason you will be asked to cough a lot to expel the mucus. If you find the coughing painful, take a deep breath, hold your hand on your incision, and forcefully expel air from your lungs.

Between two and four weeks postpartum, you can discuss a more strenuous exercise routine with your doctor, depending on how well you are recovering. An easy walking and stretching program is fine, provided you have no complications. Listening to your body and not overstressing yourself is essential. Don't do strenuous exercise. Postpone jogging, weight lifting, crunches, and other heavy-duty exercise until at least six weeks. If you start exercising too soon, you could injure yourself, and it will take even longer to recover. You could delay wound closure and increase vaginal bleeding. Doctors also advise that you don't climb stairs or drive in the first four weeks at least. This is because abdominal stiffness will make it painful to look over your shoulder, and your reflexes won't be so sharp.

At six weeks you will probably have your second postpartum checkup. If you are doing well, you can start stretching and strengthening exercises. Bear in mind, though, that it will take a while longer before you can begin abdominal strengthening exercises in order to allow your incision to fully heal. Once you and your doctor feel you are ready, you can start more high-impact and strenuous exercise. But be sure to start out slowly to avoid muscle and joint strain.

Stress Reduction

Too much stress makes weight management far more difficult. Having a baby is stressful. At times you will feel overwhelmed. It's so tempting to reach for that tub of ice cream for comfort to postpone exercise.

Exercise and a healthy diet are the best ways to ease postpartum stress. If you treat your body with respect, you will soon find that you become more resilient. As well as this, though, stress reduction cannot really be achieved without some kind of inner calm. Try for a few moments each day to sit quietly or lie down with your eyes shut. Concentrate just on your breathing and put aside other thoughts. If thoughts keep interfering, notice them and then go back to concentrating on your breathing. Find some time, even if it is just a few minutes each day, just for you. You deserve it. It's a tough job being a new mom. Take some time for peace and solitude so that you can come back to your routines refreshed and calm.

24

The Postpartum
Weight Loss Plateau

"I've lost twenty pounds since I had my baby, but now I'm stuck. I just can't lose those last ten pounds."

"I eat healthily and I exercise every day. I've been the same weight for weeks now."

Often when weight plateaus, you are closer than ever to losing weight. However, seeing your weight stay the same for weeks on end after an initial weight loss is a fact of life in the postpartum period. It is important to keep eating healthily. Trying to speed up weight loss by severely restricting your food intake is no solution—your body will recognize the reduction in calories and cling to that fat even harder.

Don't get angry with yourself. Instead, think of how far you have come. How much weight you have lost. Think about how much more energy you have now. How your clothes are starting to fit again. How much easier it is now to climb the stairs. Make a mental note of all the improvements you notice to stay motivated.

In the early months, weight plateaus can be explained by your body conserving fat stores for your baby, but if you are more than six months postpartum, you need to think about whether this is really a plateau or if you have in fact reached your natural weight. The weight your body feels comfortable at. If you are 70 pounds over what most charts recommend for your height and build, this could well be a plateau, but if you are just 10 pounds away, you might consider accepting your weight. Is it really worth punishing yourself with a stricter regime to achieve a weight that is perhaps unnatural for you?

Is This Really a Plateau?

To recognize if you are really in a plateau, think whether you are doing any strength training. Muscles weigh more than fat. That's why scales can be misleading now. You may not show a weight loss, but with muscle replacing fat, you will look a lot better. You might also want to check with your doctor if you have any condition that interferes with weight loss, such as high cholesterol, high blood pressure, diabetes, high glucose, thyroid problems, and hormonal imbalance.

Also important to consider is where your fat is stored. If it is around your middle, this is the greatest risk to your health. Fat stores accumulated here are associated with heart disease, diabetes, and certain types of cancer. And finally, take an honest look at your diet and exercise program. How much are you actually eating? Is it nutritious? Are you exercising enough?

If you are eating a balanced diet with the appropriate number of calories for your age and build, and you do regular strength training combined with aerobics, it is probable that your body has simply settled at a weight that is best for you. If this is a few pounds off your prepregnancy weight, is that really so bad? You are healthy and you have a beautiful baby to love and care for. Remember how you trusted your body during pregnancy to know what was best for you and your baby. Why not try trusting its wisdom now and accept your weight? If getting into your prepregnancy clothes is causing you anxiety, consider renewing your wardrobe.

Promoting Weight Loss When You Hit a Plateau

If, on the other hand, you really think you have reached a plateau and that you do need to lose some more weight, there are some things you can do to promote weight loss.

Consider cross training. Are you stuck in an exercise rut? Running the same number of miles every week? Swimming the same number of laps? When muscles get used to an exercise pattern, they begin to adapt. Your body becomes accustomed to a particular type of exercise and burns fewer calories doing it. To keep your calorie burn high, mix your workouts. Combine walking with cycling, or jogging with swimming, or stair climbing with aerobic classes, and so on. You could also build up the intensity of your workout. During your workout, pick up the pace for one to three minutes, then return to your normal pace for three to five minutes. Keep repeating this cycle throughout your workout. This will help you burn more calories.

Think about how active you are in your daily life. In this modern age of phones, faxes, TVs, cars, elevators, and Internet shopping, we are far less active than our moms were fifty years ago. Try to keep as active as possible during the day. If you are exercising aerobically, you may need to go for longer. Regular aerobic exercise, such as fast walking for forty-five minutes or so a few times a week, will help you burn fat. But studies have shown that exercise for forty-five to sixty minutes at least five times a week is effective for weight loss.

If weight training is not in your routine, you might consider working on your muscle strength. The less muscle you have, the fewer calories you will burn. In *Strong Women Stay Slim* (Bantam, 1998), author Miriam Nelson describes how muscles burn calories faster than fat. Women with greater muscle mass use up more calories even when they are not active. Often when moms lose weight by cutting calories and only doing aerobic exercises such as walking, they lose muscle along with fat. Each pound of muscle you lose decreases the amount you must eat to maintain your weight by 35 calories. Losing a pound of fat, on the other hand, lowers the burn by 2 calories only. The secret is to maximize fat loss while maintaining muscles. Keep working aerobically but start weight training or muscle toning exercises several times a week to build a slimmer, firmer body. If you do training with weights, make sure you have a rest day between workouts, and if possible, get a fitness trainer to develop a program for you that works the major muscles.

All the exercise in the world won't help you, though, if you are eating the wrong kinds of food. Sometimes when you start to lose weight initially, you are not as diligent as you were in the beginning. Portion sizes start to increase. Sweets creep back into your diet. You could be eating more calories than you think. Keeping a food diary and watching what you eat again will help. This does not mean severely restricting your diet. It just means making a few small changes: reducing your portion size, using skim milk, avoiding butter, having a salad daily, eating more fruit, and avoiding high-fat, high-calorie foods such as pizza and ice cream.

Remember, too, that if you want to avoid gaining the weight back again, you have to think of your healthy diet and exercise routine as a permanent part of your life style. You just can't go back to your old habits anymore unless you want to see the pounds pile back on again. Don't think of postpartum weight management as dieting and exercising to lose weight. Rather, think of it as eating and keeping active to lose weight and look toned and fit for the rest of your life.

Helpful Weight Management Review Tips

Eat a high carbohydrate diet. No, make that protein diet. Try Weight Watchers. No, try the Slim Fast drinks. Fast for one day a month. Never fast—it slows your metabolism. Never eat after 7 P.M. It doesn't matter what time of day you eat—it is what you eat that matters. Try....

The real secret to weight loss postpartum seems to be making sense of all the conflicting advice out there. For every theory about weight loss, you are bound to hear exactly the opposite. But there is a body basic you can rely on: If you want to lose weight, you have to exercise more, eat less, and preferably do both together.

Here is a summary of the most helpful tips for successful post partum weight management.

1. Make sure you keep as active as possible.
2. Combine strength training with aerobic activity.
3. Don't underestimate how much you are eating. A food diary where you record everything you eat can be really helpful. It is important to get an accurate sense of your food intake and to watch the size of your portions if you want to lose weight.
4. Don't go on very restrictive diets. Your body will cling to the fat you have if you do. You won't be getting all your nutrients, either.

5. Don't get hung up on counting calories. Make sure your diet contains a correct balance of all the nutrients you need. Concentrate on nutrient-rich foods which help you lose weight. Eat foods that will help you lose weight.

6. Don't cut out all the foods you enjoy from your diet. Just eat them in moderation. Losing weight and being miserable do not have to be the same thing.

7. The most effective way to lose weight and to keep it off is to lose it gradually and slowly—a pound or so a week if you are not breastfeeding, a pound or two a month if you are.

8. Forgive yourself. No one is perfect. So if you miss your usual workout or succumb to a Starbucks mocha with full cream, don't berate yourself and give up. Instead, acknowledge your slip—after all, you are human—and then get back on track. It's what you do most of the time that matters.

9. Stop weighing yourself. Listen to your body and how it feels. Instead of focusing on the scales, focus on exercise and eating right and feeling healthy. Permanent weight loss will follow, along with other benefits—more energy, a better night's sleep, fewer aches and pains, lower blood pressure, and being able to carry your baby up the stairs without getting out of breath.

10. Be patient. You will get there in time. Pregnancy weight gain is not permanent. You can lose it. Remember, it took your body nine months to gain the weight. It takes most women nine months to a year to lose it. And should you finally lose it, make sure you continue eating sensibly and exercising so that the weight doesn't pile back on again.

25

It's Not What
Babies Do to Your Body,
It's What They Do
to Your Life

WHILE I WAS WRITING THIS BOOK, I TOOK TIME OUT TO MEET AN OLD
friend of mine. It was while we were having coffee together that she
casually mentioned that she and her partner were planning to "start a
family."

"What do you think?" she laughs. "Will we be good parents?
Should I have a baby? Will it ruin my figure?"

"Your life will never be the same," I say quietly and calmly.

"Oh, I know," she laughs again. "No more late nights, no more
spur-of-the-moment vacations."

But this is not what I meant.

I want to tell her about being a mom, but I don't know where to
start. I want to tell her about all the things she won't read in books or
learn in her prenatal classes.

I want to tell her that a news report about an abandoned baby will
send her into inconsolable sobs. Images of malnourished children will
haunt her forever. That she can imagine nothing more terrible in life
than watching her child suffer.

I notice her designer clothes, her immaculate makeup, high heels,
and manicured nails. I want to tell her that when she is a mom she'll
be happiest in her leggings. Happy to be drooled on. Happy to have
her hair tugged. Happy to forgo her manicure if it means spending
more time with her baby.

I want to tell her that her attitude toward her career will change.
That the first day back at work will be heartbreaking. That she will

need incredible discipline to focus on the task in hand. That she will constantly worry if baby is all right.

I want to warn her that her life will never have routine and order again. That the most carefully laid plans can be disrupted at a moment's notice when baby refuses to eat or sleep or gets sick. That, however brilliant she is about making decisions at work, when it comes to decisions about her child she will always anxiously wonder if she is really doing the best.

I'd like to tell her that she might get her figure back. But I want her to understand that her appearance, her own life just won't seem so important when baby is born. That she would willingly throw herself in front of a train if it meant saving her child. That she'll still have dreams, but her child's hopes and dreams will be her passion now.

I want her to know that she will come to respect and cherish the memories of her pregnancy. That she will look fondly at her stretch marks and scars. That gaining a few pounds or losing a few pounds won't matter so much to her anymore.

Her relationship will change, but not in the way she thinks. As she watches her partner cherish and care for the baby with tenderness, her love will grow. She will discover love again for the most unromantic reasons.

I want her to know that she will think about the world differently. She'll want it to be a better place for her baby. That she will worry about nuclear war and global warming. That she'll fret about drunk driving, cigarettes, alcohol, swearing, and teenage sex.

I want to articulate for my friend the sheer joy she will experience when her baby smiles at her for the first time. I want to capture for her how incredible it is to watch her baby discover life. How she will see life again through her newborn's eyes. How every day will have magic in it.

I want her to feel the joy that is so great it will make her cry.

My friend looks at me, puzzled.

"You're crying," she says.

"You won't ever regret it," I say firmly. Then I close my eyes and say a prayer for every woman who discovers that most cherished and blessed of callings—that of being a mom.

It's not so much what babies do to your body, but what they do to your life. Postpartum bodily changes are only just the beginning of the many changes motherhood brings in your life.

Lack of Sleep

> "I really knew things had changed when my baby finally began to sleep for more than four hours and I considered sleeping from midnight to five A.M. sleeping through the night. I also noticed that the quality of my sleep changed. My sleep was light. I was anxious about my baby. He might need me. The slightest murmur and I would be wide awake in mommy mode."

One of the most noticeable changes postpartum is usually in the number of hours you sleep. Lack of sleep is also one of the biggest threats to postpartum weight loss in the first postpartum months and maybe even years. You may have heard how Margaret Thatcher or Oprah Winfrey can get by on four hours' sleep a night, but for the great majority of us, less than six hours' sleep a night is not enough. Adults need about six to eight hours a night to function efficiently; some of us need even more. Your baby needs an average of sixteen hours and toddlers twelve. We all have a sleep quota that we need. Your baby is probably getting it, but you are not, if your nights are filled with crying, rocking, and diapering, and your days with feeding, crying, rocking, and diapering.

Every new mom at some time or other will feel that she really needs more sleep. Moms who don't get enough sleep are more likely to overeat and consume high-sugar and high-fat drinks, according to sleep researcher James Horne, author of *Why We Sleep* (Oxford University Press, 1989). If you can't energize yourself with rest, you turn to quick energy (high-calorie) food. If you are tired, you are also far more likely to skip exercise. Fatigue is a major factor in postpartum weight gain.

"Sleep deprivation can interfere with weight loss, and cause exhaustion and severe depression," writes Colleen Sundermeyer (*I Want My Body Back*, Perigee, 1998, p. 107). Sundermeyer explains how sleep is biologically necessary for weight loss. Your metabolism slows down when you sleep, but about an hour before arising, growth hormone is released, and this stimulates fat burning. Growth hormone is released during the day, randomly and after exercise. If you are not getting enough sleep, you won't be releasing enough growth hormone, and this will stop you burning fat.

It is going to be a difficult juggling act to get a good night's sleep, but there are things you can do to help you cope better and improve the quality of your sleep. Nap whenever and wherever you can. Nap when baby naps. Try to nap for at least thirty minutes, but no more than two hours, to wake feeling refreshed. Eat healthily. Certain foods you eat, such as those high in sugar, can overload your system and make it difficult for you to fall asleep. Alcohol, chocolate, and coffee and tea are also sleep robbers, so try to avoid them before bedtime. Healthy eating habits promote sleep and weight loss. Exercise will also make sure your body is tired when you go to bed. Don't exercise in the evening, though, this will interfere with your sleep. If you can manage it, go to sleep earlier rather than rising late. This is easier for your body clock.

Your Relationship

There are three of you now. You might find yourself looking back at those carefree days when you just had each other to love and care for. Afternoons at the movies, dinners out, and all those fun things just the two of you used to do are all in the past. Your life is organized around baby's timetable. It is very hard to be spontaneous anymore. As discussed earlier, sex is different, too. Getting in the mood can be a problem for physical and emotional reasons. But it doesn't stop there. Even if you are in the mood, finding time and getting some privacy can be a challenge.

There is adjusting to do when two becomes three, but soon you won't be able to imagine life together without baby. She is a part of you both. The part that makes you whole.

Your Work

You will certainly find that you have a changed attitude toward work.

Many of the women I talked to said that having a baby put the crisis and challenges of work into perspective. You have other priorities now. Others said that work became even more important for a sense of self. Some intended to go back to work but found themselves unable to leave baby when their maternity leave ended. A few said that they resented the fact that they had to go back to work out of financial necessity. Several said that having a baby made them rethink their career entirely. Others started new careers. Some decided to work from home. Whether working or staying at home, it was clear that feelings of guilt about working or not working figured strongly for both stay-at-home and working moms.

Your Friends

One of the saddest changes when you have a baby may be that your old circle of friends gradually diminishes. True friendships usually survive, but many won't. I tried to avoid becoming a baby bore with friends who had no children, but I found that I naturally gravitated toward other moms. I wanted to talk about my baby. I wanted to compare notes with other moms. In the early months I joined a first-time moms' group. I was desperate for mom pals. I made instant friendships. When you become a mom, you will become part of the mommy club. The membership is for life. Of course, for a friendship to last, there have to be other things in common apart from children. But even to this day, whenever I meet new friends, it's so much easier to break the ice if they have children, too.

Your Family

Motherhood may change the way you look at your own parents. They were like you once, too. They had many of the same struggles and sacrifices to make. There is new appreciation of what they did for you. And if your relationship with your parents was conflicted, there might be a greater tolerance and understanding. On the other hand, you may be determined not to repeat the mistakes you believe your parents made when they brought you up. Either way, motherhood will make you think about how your own childhood and how you were brought up shaped who you are.

Your Time

Time may suddenly becomes very precious when you become a parent. You cherish every moment. Weeks, months, and years fly by so quickly. Many of the parents I talked to said their lives had become one big juggling act, with never enough time for anything.

Your World View

You could find yourself becoming more compassionate. Everyone was an innocent, vulnerable, impressionable baby once. The suffering of innocent children around the world could send a knife through your heart. You may also become more critical of the society you live in. The values your community hold. As a mother, you just won't want your impressionable child to be subjected to the messages of violence our culture celebrates, or those of sex and money, either.

Your Life

You'll probably think differently about your own life, too. You might become more aware of your own mortality. Who will look after your baby and love him if something happened to you? You could end up a little more anxious about everything, but at the same time you could also become more tolerant and patient. You may discover a love so strong it can bring tears to your eyes. You might also develop this amazing ability to do a hundred things at once. You might emerge from the experience of childbirth more mature and responsible. After all, you have a child to love and discipline. You could also discover how firm and authoritative you can be, and this helps all aspects of your life. You won't suffer in silence anymore if you or your child has been unjustly treated. Perhaps the biggest change, though, is that you could become less self-centered. For the first time in your life, you know without a doubt that you would sacrifice your own life for the sake of someone else—your child.

Your Body

Having a baby will probably change your body. Whether this is for the better or the worse is largely up to you—what you eat and how active you are. How you manage your unique life.

It may also change how you feel about your body. After baby, you might be less inhibited about your body. You may also feel more accepting and appreciative of your body and understand how remarkable it is. How it really does know what is best for you. How motherhood offers you the chance to learn to live in and accept the body that is right for you. That we are not all meant to be a size 8. That your health and baby's health is far more important than how much you weigh.

Motherhood can change your body, your life, and your mind about a great many things. It is important, though, not to overromanticize the notion of "mommy." The fact that a woman has a baby does not mean that all her attitudes will immediately become bigger and more compassionate. Plenty of women retain narrow attitudes after childbirth. What makes the difference is not just going through the biological process, but being open to the experience. Becoming spiritually aware, and paying attention to the changes.

These changes may seem overwhelming at times, but if you are open to them, in time you will see that they enrich your life in ways you could barely have imagined possible.

26

I Want to Do It Again

"There's really not much point losing weight. I want to get pregnant again."

"I had fifteen pounds to lose from my last baby. I'm pregnant again. How much weight should I put on?"

"How long should I wait till I can get pregnant again?"

"Do I want to put my body through that another time?"

You've just put your body through the most incredible of transformations. Coming to terms with your new body image is still a work in progress. Then one morning you look at your baby. She is growing fast. Too heavy now for you to carry for long periods of time. Too active to sit contentedly in your lap and gaze adoringly in your eyes. Too big now to nestle in the crook of your arm and sleep. You forget all the sleepless nights, the endless diaper changes, the endless crying. You forget all about the extra pounds you might have gained on your hips, the softer stomach you may have. You remember only the gentle moments. How huge those inky eyes were. How tiny the hands and feet were. You remember the thrill of being handed your newborn for the first time.

You want to have another baby.

Getting Pregnant the Second Time

"When are you going to give your little boy a brother or a sister?"

It might not be too long before you start hearing this from friends and family. For some couples having a second child is easy. For others it is not. Your chances of getting pregnant do not improve after each pregnancy. The average time is still six months, regardless of how many children you have had. If you have been trying longer than a year, it is wise to go and check with your doctor.

You will be older when you try to have a second child, and your lifestyle will have probably changed. These factors will affect how long it takes you to conceive. Some couples may have real trouble getting pregnant; this is called secondary infertility. For every twelve couples trying to get pregnant, six have already conceived at least once. This condition can be just as frustrating and agonizing as primary infertility, with the exception that because you already have a baby, you won't get as much sympathy.

In almost all cases of secondary infertility, experts can identify the cause, and they can help about 75 percent of couples to conceive. Carrying excessive weight, being extremely underweight, excessive exercise, or eating a poor diet are all causes of infertility, whether primary or secondary. If you want to have another baby, it is more important than ever to pay attention to sensible diet, exercise, and weight management.

How Long Should I Wait Between Babies?

As soon as you get your menstrual cycle back, you can conceive. This can be in a matter of weeks after birth, or six months to a year if you are breastfeeding.

The advice given about the space between babies and when your body is ready will vary from doctor to doctor. Some say six months, others a year, others eighteen months. Advice given by psychologists that takes children's mental and emotional well-being into account will be different again. A few decades ago, three years was the recommended time. Between one and five years is now thought to be best.

Whatever space you have between babies, there will be some kind of stress. There is no magic formula for a conflict-free family. This is reassuring for those of you who want to have a baby sooner, or for those who have an unplanned but welcome second pregnancy.

When you're thinking about a second child, the best time is when you feel ready to cope with it. Pregnancy and childbirth, as you know, are demanding. It's wise to make sure you are in the best emotional and physical health before you think about baby number two.

How does your body feel? Have you lost most of the weight gained? Have you and your partner adjusted to family life well? Is your relationship strong? Has your closeness and intimacy returned? If you had the baby blues, have they gone away? What about work? Have you resolved problems with day care? Are you still tired? After baby is weaned and you are getting more sleep, you should be feeling more energetic. If you are still feeling constantly tired, you need to look into that before considering another baby. Have you gotten treatment for postpartum discomforts such as backache, incontinence, hemorrhoids, varicose veins?

As far as body management is concerned, the best time to conceive a second baby is probably about a year later. By this time your body will have fully recovered. A year also gives you longer to manage your weight and return to your prepregnancy weight.

Why Losing Postpartum Weight Is Important Before You Conceive Again

You might think it's not worth bothering to lose weight if you want to get pregnant again. Well, it is. Any excess weight you carry when you get pregnant again will not be considered baby fat. It is just plain old fat. The weight you are when you get pregnant will be the weight you must start gaining from. Unless you are very overweight, you should not gain less than the recommended twenty-five to thirty-five pounds to ensure a healthy delivery. You cannot diet when you are pregnant.

If you still have weight to lose from your first baby, you'll probably consider limiting your overall weight gain in your second. Say you are ten pounds overweight—you decide to gain ten pounds less this time around. It just isn't that easy, though. Before you know it, you have twenty pounds to lose after baby number two.

If you want to have a baby, the best thing you can do for yourself is to be strict about getting to a weight you are comfortable with and that is healthy before you get pregnant. Even five pounds extra will make a difference. If you don't lose excess weight now, you risk an accumulation of weight with each baby that is likely to become permanent.

Diet and Exercise Prepregnancy

(For advice about prepregnancy diet and exercise, see Chapter One.)

If you want to get pregnant again, good nutrition is essential. If you still have weight to lose, try to lose it by increasing your activity levels and eating a healthy diet with fewer calories. Don't severely restrict your food intake. Getting your body back into condition before pregnancy is important, too. Concentrate on strengthening the muscles that are most strained by pregnancy—the abdominals, the pelvic floor muscles that support your bowel and uterus, and your back muscles.

Is It Different the Second Time Around?

Not really. There might be some differences, but the major characteristics of pregnancy remain the same. If you had morning sickness, you'll probably get it again, regardless of the sex of your baby. If you got depressed after baby, you'll feel depressed again, unless you have found solutions to emotional conflicts.

As far as weight gain is concerned, you'll probably find that you gain about the same amount of weight. Many women I talked to said that they gained nearly the same each time, regardless of whether they ate and exercised. Don't use this as an excuse to eat junk food and become a couch potato, though. Exercising and eating right during pregnancy are still essential for the health of you and baby-to-be, regardless of what your body decides it must gain.

You will usually show sooner with your next baby. If you began to show in the fifth month, you could show in the third or fourth now. This is because your abdominal muscles are less resilient. Aches and pains also tend to be more frequent with the next baby, simply because your body has less support and is looser the second time around. Looser conditions around the uterus and birth canal mean that you might have more Braxton-Hicks contractions (false contractions). A thinner uterus that has been stretched once might also mean that you feel your baby kick sooner. (Or this could just be because you are familiar with the feeling and know what to look for.) Hemorrhoids, varicose veins, stress incontinence, and other pregnancy delights tend to get worse with each baby. If you had gestational diabetes the first time around, you may get it again.

Lightening, when your baby's head drops down into the pelvis area, may not occur in your second pregnancy. The length of your pregnancy will probably mirror your first. Labor definitely tends to be faster, but many women say it is more intense and painful. Just because you had a cesarean section the first time around does not mean you have to have one again.

In the postpartum period, contractions of the uterus, called after-pains, tend to be more vigorous and painful as the uterus has to work harder to contract second time around. Milk comes in earlier and breastfeeding is less uncomfortable and traumatic. Your milk production factory is much more efficient the second time around. If you had a cesarean, your recovery rate will probably be faster.

Is It Harder to Get Back in Shape?

It's no harder to return to a healthy weight postpartum, unless, of course you had excess weight to lose from your first baby. You'll probably have to work out harder to get abdominal tone back, though. The same applies for your pelvic floor muscles.

All in all, though, a second pregnancy won't really have any more of an effect on your body than the first. You might be reluctant to inflict more damage on your breasts, your vagina, your stomach, and your back, but the truth is that a second pregnancy, or a third or a fourth pregnancy, won't really make much of a difference. You have already been stretched. A second child won't stretch you any more. Your first baby changed your body permanently. Your other babies work with what they have.

Will You Feel Different?

Friends and families won't make such a fuss over you this time around, but you will feel less anxious and able to enjoy your second pregnancy more. After all, you have done it before. You know what to expect. You'll probably savor every moment because you know how quickly time flies between pregnancy and your baby becoming a toddler. You realize how unique, fleeting, and special this time in your life is, and how very rewarding it can be. On the other hand, you may feel guilty that with your first-born to tend to you can't pay as much attention to this pregnancy as you would like.

You'll probably feel nervous about how your firstborn will react. You'll wonder if you can ever love your second baby as much as the first. You'll wonder how you will find time to do anything. You'll wonder where you will find the energy. You'll wonder how much time you will get to spend alone with your partner. You'll wonder if you can afford another baby. You'll wonder why after months of getting your body back in some kind of shape, you have gone and spoiled it all again. You'll wonder if you will ever get your figure back. You'll wonder how long it will take to lose the weight. You'll wonder why on earth you are putting your body through this. You'll wonder why on earth you have decided to have another baby.

But when your newborn arrives, you forget all the aches and pains, the weight gain, and other bodily changes. You discover that there is plenty of room in your heart for two. You realize once again what a blessing and a celebration having a baby is. And as you watch your children grow, you'll wonder how on earth you could ever have imagined life without any of them.

Afterword

IF YOU THINK YOU WILL NEVER LOSE YOUR PREGNANCY WEIGHT, TAKE A deep breath and remind yourself of these basics about postpartum weight loss.

- You can lose weight by increasing your exercise levels and eating more fruit and vegetables and less fat and sugar.
- Most of us won't lose the weight right away. It will take a good nine months to a year. Be patient. Slow and gradual weight loss is the best way to get in shape.

You may be in for a surprise, though, when you finally reach your target weight.... Nine months after the birth of my baby boy, at a well-woman checkup, I was weighed. A little hesitant, I stepped on the scales. I was amazed to discover that I was a pound under my prepregnancy weight. I had done it. I had lost my baby fat.

But what surprised me more was that it really didn't seem a big deal anymore. I was pleased, but not as thrilled as I thought I would be.

I have changed since I had my baby. What gives me a thrill now is not fitting into a size 8 pair of jeans, but waking my baby up in the morning, watching him smile, watching him grow. What gets me excited is talking about having another baby. Many people say that when you have a baby you lose your freedom, but I found a new sense of freedom. Freedom from the scales. Of course I still didn't want to be overweight. But these things don't define who I am anymore. My health, my family, my friends, my work are what give me joy.

Put the whole business of how much you weigh in perspective. Sensible weight management during pregnancy and postpartum is important. Excess weight will affect your self-esteem. Looking after your body and managing your weight is one of the most important things you can do for yourself as a mother and as a woman. But if there is a little sagging here and there, a little softness, maybe even a few extra pounds, doesn't your baby make it all worth it?

Resources

Organizations

ANRED (Anorexia Nervosa and Related Eating Disorders, Inc.) a Eugene, OR, educational association (www.anred.com)
Tel: (541) 344-1144

NEDO (National Eating Disorders Organization) Tulsa, OK
Tel: (918) 481-4044

AABA (American Anorexia Bulimia Association), New York.
Tel: (212) 575-6200

American College of Nurse-Midwives
818 Connecticut Ave., NW, Suite 900
Washington, DC 20006

American College of Obstetricians and Gynecologists
409 12th Street, SW
Washington, DC 20024

American Council on Exercise
5820 Oberlin Drive, Suite 102
San Diego, CA 92121

Depression After Delivery
PO Box 1282
Morrisville, PA 19067
Tel (800) 944-4773
www.behavenet.com

La Leche League for Breastfeeding
9616 Minneapolis Ave.
Franklin Park, IL 60131
Tel: (800) LA LECHE

Postpartum Education Hotline
Tel: (805) 564-3888

Sideline National Support Network—
a support group for women who are bedridden during pregnancy
PO Box 1808
Laguna Beach, CA 92652
Tel: (714) 497-2265

Web Sites

HUNDREDS OF WEB SITES ON PREGNANCY WITH CHAT, LINKS, information, and advice exist for you to investigate. Here are a few:

A fun site for targeting the specific stage of your fetus's development: *www.storksite.com*

An online baby registry where you can post a photo of your baby:
www.babytalkandshop.com

An interesting site that covers a range of pregnancy and postpartum topics:
www.babycenter.com

Advice, interviews, and information about parenting:
www.parenttime.com
www.parentsplace.com

Expert pregnancy and baby advice: *www.babycenter.com*

Suggested Reading

American Baby Magazine: For Expectant and New Parents. Magazine published monthly by Primedia Inc., 249 West 17th Street, New York, NY 10011

Balch, James, and Balch, Phyllis. Prescription for Nutritional Healing: A Practical A–Z Reference to Drug-Free Remedies Using Vitamins, Minerals, Herbs and Food Supplements. New York, Avery Publishing, 1997

Behan, Eileen. Eat Well, Lose Weight While Breastfeeding: The Complete Nutrition Book for Nursing Mothers. New York, Villard Books, 1992

Blunt, Stavia. Shaping Up During and After Pregnancy. Chichester, UK, Summersdale, 1997

Brasner, Shari E. Advice from a Pregnant Obstetrician. New York, Harper Collins, 1998

Brumberg, Joan Jacobs. The Body Project: An Intimate History of American Girls. New York, Vintage, 1997

Butler, Joan Marie. Fit and Pregnant: The Pregnant Woman's Guide to Exercise. New York, Acorn, 1996

Cheung, Theresa Francis. A Break in Your Cycle: The Medical and Emotional Causes and Effects of Amenorrhea. New York, Wiley, 1998

Eiger, Marvin, and Wendkos Olds, Sally. The Complete Book of Breastfeeding. New York, Workman, 1987

Eisenberg, Arlene, Murkoff, Heidi, and Hathaway, Sandee. What to Expect When You're Expecting. New York, Workman, 1996

Eisenberg, Arlene, Murkoff, Heidi, and Hathaway, Sandee. What to Expect the First Year. New York, Workman, 1996

Erick, M. No More Morning Sickness: A Survival Guide for Pregnant Women. New York, Penguin, 1993

Fit Pregnancy: For the Whole Nine Months and Beyond. Magazine published quarterly by Shape Magazine, 21100 Erwin St., Woodland Hills, CA 91367

Gillespie, Clark. Your Pregnancy Month by Month: A Comprehensive Guide and Personal Diary. New York, Harper Collins, 1992

Horne, James. Why We Sleep. Oxford University Press, Oxford, 1989

Huggins, Kathleen, and Ziedrich, Linda. The Nursing Mother's Guide to Weaning. Massachusetts, Harvard Common Press, 1994

Iovine, Vicki. The Girlfriends' Guide to Surviving the First Year of Motherhood. New York, Perigee, 1997

Iovine, Vicki. The Girlfriends' Guide to Pregnancy. New York, Pocket Books, 1996

Iovine, Vicki. The Girlfriends' Guide to Pregnancy: Daily Diary. New York, Pocket Books, 1996

Kleiman, Karen, and Raskin, Valerie. This Isn't What I Expected: Overcoming Postpartum Depression. New York, Bantam, 1994

La Leche League International. The Womanly Art of Breastfeeding. New York, Plume, 1997

Lerner, Harriot. The Mother Dance: How Children Change Your Life. New York, Harper Collins, 1998

Louden, Jennifer. The Pregnant Woman's Comfort Book: A Self-Nurturing Guide to Your Emotional Well-Being During Pregnancy and Early Motherhood. San Francisco, Harper, 1995

Manuel, Alvarez, and Feiden, Karyn. *Recovering from Cesarean Section*. New York, Harper, 1993

Marshall, Connie. *From Here to Maternity: A Complete Pregnancy Guide*. Minden, N.V., Conmar, 1997

Misri, Shaila. *Shouldn't I Be Happy? Emotional Problems of Pregnant and Postpartum Women*. New York, Free Press, 1995

Mungeam, Frank. *A Guy's Guide to Pregnancy: Preparing for Parenthood Together*. Hillsboro, OR, Beyond Words, 1998

Nelson, Miriam. *Strong Women Stay Slim*. New York, Bantam, 1998

Noble, Elizabeth. *Essential Exercises for the Childbearing Year: A Guide to Health and Comfort Before and After Your Baby Is Born*. Harwich, MA, New Life Images, 1995

Northrup, Christiane. *Women's Bodies, Women's Wisdom*. New York, Bantam, 1995

Olkin, Sylvia Klein. *Positive Pregnancy Fitness: A Total Approach to a More Comfortable and Easier Birth*. New York, Avery, 1987

Olkin, Sylvia Klein. *Positive Parenting Fitness: A Total Approach to Caring for the Physical and Emotional Needs of Your New Fmaily*. New York, Avery, 1987

Parents Magazine published monthly by Gruner and Jahr USA Publishing, 375 Lexington Avenue, New York NY 10017

Pipher, Mary. *Hunger Pains: The Modern Woman's Tragic Quest for Thinness*. New York, Ballantine, 1995

Rako, Susan. *The Hormone of Desire: The Truth about Sexuality, Menopause and Testosterone*. New York, Harmony, 1996

Robin, Peggy. *Bottle-Feeding Without Guilt: A Reassuring Guide for Loving Parents*. Rocklin, CA, Prima, 1996

Roth, Geneen. *Feeding the Hungry Heart: The Experience of Compulsive Eating*. New York, Plume, 1993

Scattergood, Emma. *Mother and Baby Exercise: An Easy Program to Take You Through Pregnancy*. London, Ward Lock, 1995

Shannon, Jacqueline. *The New Mother's Body Book*. Chicago, Contemporary, 1994

Shapiro, Jerrold Lee. *When Men Are Pregnant: Needs and Concerns of Expectant Fathers*. New York, Delta, 1987

Siegal, Paula M. *The Next Nine Months: A Guide to Your Body After Giving Birth*. New York, Penguin, 1996

Somer, Elizabeth. *Nutrition for a Healthy Pregnancy: The Complete Guide to Eating Before, During and After Your Pregnancy*. New York, Henry Holt, 1995

Sundermeyer, Colleen A. *I Want My Body Back: Nutrition and Weight Loss for Mothers*. New York, Perigee, 1998

Thurston, Jeffrey. *1000 Questions about Your Pregnancy*. Arlington, TX, Summit, 1997

Trexler, Sandra, and Trexler, Michael. *Bye Bye Baby Fat: Reshaping the New Mother Mind and Body*. Fort Worth, TX, Summit, 1994

Wright, Elizabeth. *The New Mother's Survival Guide*. Nashville, TN, Cumberland House, 1997

YMCA of the USA with Thomas Hanlon. *Fit for Two: The Official YMCA Prenatal Exercise Guide*. Champaign, IL, Human Kinetics, 1995

Index

A

Abdomen
    after C-section, 129–130
    during pregnancy, 22, 26, 99
    exercise for, 206, 210
    postpartum, 122, 124, 131–132
Aerobic exercise
    during pregnancy, 87
    postpartum, 209, 219
Age
    pregnancy and, 178–179
    weight gain and, 105
    weight loss and, 179–180
Alcohol, avoiding, 6, 62, 67, 199
Anorexia. *See* Eating disorders
Aspirin, avoiding, 69

B

Baby
    development of, in utero, 20, 24, 27
    predicting birth weight of, 35–36
    ways of carrying, in utero, 36–37
Backache
    during pregnancy, 22, 80, 91–92
    postpartum, 127
Beauty, changing standards of, 11–12
Bed rest, 76
Belly. *See* Abdomen
Biking, 87
Biotin, 58
Bleeding, postpartum, 128, 207
BMI (body mass index), 8, 172
    chart, 9
Body image
    postpartum anxiety about, 143–146,
        149–153
    rethinking one's, 10–14, 99–101,
        171–174
Bottle-feeding, weight loss and, 190–191
Braxton-Hicks contractions, 232
Breastfeeding, 138–139
    exercise and, 213–214
    fat loss and, 120
    menstrual cycle and, 118
    nutrition and, 193–203
    preparation for, 137
    sexual relations and, 155, 156
    uterine shrinkage and, 122
    weight loss and, 184, 186–191,
        196–197
    see also Breasts
Breasts
    at delivery, 137–138
    during pregnancy, 18, 21, 25, 98,
        135–137
    postpartum, 140, 156
    weaning and, 139
    see also Breastfeeding
Bulimia. *See* Eating disorders

C

C-section
    exercise after, 182, 214–215
    recovery from, 129–130, 192–193
    sexual relations after, 156
Caffeine, avoiding, 6, 62, 199
Calcium, 58, 60, 65–66, 68, 195
    leg cramps and, 95–96
Caloric requirements
    of breastfeeding, 188, 193, 197
    of pregnancy, 63–67
Carbohydrates, 56, 198–199
Cesarean section. *See* C-section
Cigarettes, avoiding, 6, 67
Colostrum, 136, 137, 138
Conception. *See* Fertility
Constipation
    during pregnancy, 23, 73–74, 80
    postpartum, 124, 126
Copper, 58, 65
Couvade syndrome, 165–166
Cramps, during pregnancy, 22, 95–96
Cravings, 77–78

D

Depression After Delivery (DAD), 143
Diabetes, 75–76, 232
Diastasis, 124, 125
Diet